SHE'S HOT, HE'S NOT

Just One More Thing That Makes Men and Women Different

SHE'S HOT, HE'S NOT

Just One More Thing That Makes Men and Women Different

By Carolyn Y. Billups

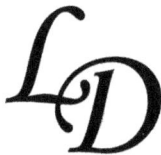

LD

LavalDreams
PUBLISHING

ISBN-13: 978-0-9851546-3-9

Book editing by Sharon Hogg and Laval Belle

Book cover design by Babypie Publishing

Book layout and print setup by Babypie Publishing

Author photo by Jonathan Solomon, Freshh Photography

LavalDreams
8549 Wilshire
Beverly Hills, CA 90211

Visit our website at: www.lavaldream.com

Published & Printed in the United States of America

Dedication

This book is dedicated to the honor and loving memory of my parents, Joseph and Kazuyo, who lived a phenomenal life of nobility, purity, goodness, and virtue.

This book is also dedicated to my beautiful daughters Miki, Jeneice, and Rose; my fabulous niece Natasha "Pumpkin"; and my lovely sister Sachi

This book was written in mind for all the precious women around the world who are *hot* in more ways than one.

We are blessed and highly favored!

This book was written for the benefit of men everywhere,

Those who think they know all about women,

Those who want to know more about women,

And those who have no clue about women.

Table of Contents

Introduction   9

Chapter 1: What Are Hot Flashes?   13

Chapter 2: Uncovering The Heat   31

Chapter 3: He Doesn't Get It   43

Chapter 4: When The Real One Hits   63

Chapter 5: Freezing The Moment   71

Chapter 6: 95 And Flashing   91

Chapter 7: Putting Out The Flame   99

Chapter 8: Life In Different Climates   117

Acknowledgements & References   125

Special Thanks   129

Introduction

After experiencing my first hot flash, I suddenly knew exactly what my mother went through some twenty years ago. Until now, I had no idea why she would strip down naked and slip into a muumuu (a loose dress originating from Hawaii) every time she came home from running errands, or keep a damp wash cloth in the freezer to press against her neck and forehead several times a day, leave her bedroom window cracked open about an inch all year round, or insist on wearing thin short-sleeved tops even in the coldest of winters. She would freeze everyone out by turning off the heat in the winter! Mom would turn off the thermostat and dad would turn it on to 80 degrees. My mother would come back and turn it off again screaming, "Who turned this up?" And my father would sneak back and crank it up to 90 degrees. This back and forth battle would go on several times until my mother would inevitably win leaving my father no choice but to sit in front of the oven with its door open trying to stay warm. I called this the "Battle of the Thermostat." I kid you not - he would be wearing his heaviest robe with a knit cap on his bald head rubbing his hands together while sitting directly in front of the open oven set at 400 degrees in one of those high-back dining room chairs. The first time I saw it, I fell out laughing. I have to admit it was brilliant! My mother couldn't do anything but scoff at him.

Then **IT** happened! On January 6, 2011, at an upscale restaurant celebrating the one-year anniversary of my father's passing, I felt it - the uncontrollable surge of formidable heat that seemed to come out of nowhere and no amount of fanning could make it subside, until finally, this unpredictable burst passed after what seemed an eternity. I'd never felt anything like this before. This surprise intruder entered from somewhere deep within my body, moved into my chest, up through my neck, and to my head until sweat was pouring profusely. My glasses steamed up like a sauna. This was a very eye-opening and embarrassing moment for me. I was shocked and disappointed at the same time and instinctively knew exactly what had just happened, but wasn't prepared and had no idea how to react.

This uncontrolled physiological episode and the many that followed propelled me to write this book. I want people to know - men, women, and even children - what women go through physically, emotionally, mentally, and even spiritually when our bodies go through these life changes. It's scary, ugly, difficult, inconvenient, painful, frustrating, time consuming, embarrassing, and beautiful at the same time.

Women, I hope this book helps you get through this tough life phase. It's not enough that we have to endure the physical pain of becoming a woman at an early age with our monthly cycle and tolerate that pain for several decades, but then to go through yet another set of physical challenges in our latter years is almost heartbreaking. We can do this and I want to show you how!

Men, you'll be provided a better understanding of what it's like for women experiencing hot flashes. The mystery behind why she is always hot or tosses and turns at night and doesn't want to be bothered with you, why she is short-tempered or tunes you out will be dispelled. It's not because she's mean or spiteful, but her body becomes extremely hot, which causes her to lose momentary focus and concentration in her thinking. When it passes, she is back to her normal self much like Jekyll and Hyde. This may be laughable, but on a serious note can be frustrating to all parties involved. There's a physiological aspect to hot flashes that will be addressed later in this book to uncover the mystery and complexity of this temporary and natural condition. Having this knowledge will hopefully give you the comfort and understanding you need to go through this time of life more smoothly and patiently with your loved one. Remember she's hot, you're not.

CHAPTER 1

WHAT ARE HOT FLASHES?

GROWING UP IN JAPAN

My parents, Joseph "Joe" Burgess and Kazuyo "Kay" Burgess, met in Iwakuni, Japan, my mother's homeland, while my father was serving in the U.S. Navy. They married and had two daughters, my sister Sachi and myself. We were born in Sasebo, Japan. My sister and I had an eventful childhood growing up in Japan where we lived for ten years spending much of our time with my mother's family.

My mother was the adventurous type so we went somewhere exciting almost every weekend with our aunts, uncles, and cousins. Our maternal grandmother, who lived nearby, often accompanied us on our excursions. She was the wisest and kindest woman I ever met, and I soon came to realize just how much my own mother was a lot like her.

My mother was a homemaker devoted to her family. She prepared home-cooked meals every single day. As a strong-willed woman, she was also very industrious and innovative. Mom sewed and knit all of our clothes and grew fresh vegetables in the garden out back. She enjoyed her quiet time as an avid reader, in both English and Japanese literature, and was a lover of classical music. She was lots of fun and loved to laugh. Though small in stature, she had this big, loud laugh and a huge smile to match.

My father was always away at work on Westpac (known as Western Pacific deployment where U.S. naval ships and vessels carrying U.S. military service members are sent out to sea on six to twelve month assignments) nine months out of every year during our ten-year residency in Japan, making it *impossible* to spend daily quality time with him growing up. When he came home for a few short days or even hours, the time we spent together was precious and priceless. We would be all over him like cotton candy. There were times when my sister and I didn't get to see him. This happened when he was granted leave for just a few hours and had to return back to the ship before it set sail again. By the time he came home, my sister and I would already be asleep in bed and he'd leave before we awakened the next morning. For my father, just being able to see his two girls and kiss us on the forehead was worth making the short trip. Dad was a hard-working family man with an excellent work ethic. He was a proud provider for his family, loved my mother very much, and was the best Father anyone could have. Everything he did was for us - his "chipmunks." That's what he called my sister and I. Even my mother referred to us as "chipmunks" from time to time. Every dime my father earned was given to my mother. She in turn managed their finances very well and we lacked for nothing. As children, we were not spoiled, but had everything we needed. I always thought we were rich!

My parents were the best cooks in the whole world. My father was a Steward in the military and spent his days in the Galley as a Cook. He wasn't just any cook but gained the reputation of being the best cook and was soon serving Captains and Admirals. He taught my mother how to cook Western food. As a native of Japan, all my mother knew, in terms of food, was from the Orient or Far East. For example, she never tasted or even heard of peanut butter until she met my father. Peanut butter didn't exist in Japan at that time. My mother had a competitive spirit, and soon mastered everything my father taught her to cook. I can't tell you who was the better cook between the two, but I can tell you I had the best of both worlds.

I mean that in every way. My parents were the best parents in the world to me. Of course, I didn't realize this until becoming an adult. As a child, I often thought my mother was the meanest person on the earth and my father was always the nicest dad who ever lived. This is because he was away so much that my mother had to take on the responsibility of being the mom and the dad of our family. Not until I had children of my own did my mother reveal how she did not want to be the disciplinarian. When it came time to scold us, she always wanted to be able to say, "Wait till your father gets home!" Instead, she had to do what was uncomfortable for her by taking the reins and playing both roles of parents in order to give my sister and I the discipline we needed. I applaud her for that.

My school years were unintentionally but quite evenly divided. I attended first through sixth grade in Hakata, Japan at a Dependent school (an American school for children of military service members and parents employed overseas). After that, we relocated to Sasebo, Japan for the next four years where I attended seventh through tenth grade at another Dependent school - Ernest J. King School. My experiences in both locations were fun and memorable. In Hakata, we were able to spend the majority of our time with my mother's side of the family because this is where they also lived. We were very close-knit and celebrated all our birthdays and holidays at our home where my mother always prepared a feast. We often traveled together to all of the touristy hot spots in the area and in the surrounding cities during those six long and marvelous years. Then in 1972, when we relocated to

Sasebo, which was three hours away, we saw less of our Japanese family. Our regular visits were reduced to holidays and special occasions, which made me very sad. It was hard even coordinating summer and winter vacations in between school terms because our summer vacations lasted three months while our Japanese cousins were only off for one month and vise versa for the winter vacations.

Life in Sasebo was different, but in a good way. It was exciting and brought to us a welcomed change. We were older and that alone elevated us to the next level. We made new friends, shared exciting adventures, and created a fresh chapter of awesome experiences. Attending E.J. King School was a grand experience. This is where we met our friends for life. The school was small with approximately two hundred students, grades one through twelve. My sister's graduating class had six seniors. Wow, right?!

I loved growing up in Japan. It was the highlight of my childhood years. The culture, the food, the people, the places all made my experiences there fun and memorable.

MOVING TO THE U.S.

On June 10, 1976, our family left Japan right after my sister graduated from high school and we relocated to San Diego, California. My father's tour of duty with the U.S. Navy had been completed and we could no longer stay in Japan as dependents of the U.S. Military. It was a sad time for us because Japan had become our home. The United States had become a foreign place to my sister and I - a mysterious land, unchartered territory, and unfamiliar ground. What would we do there? How would we interact? Would we fit in or be outcasts? What would it be like to live in America?

This was a whole new experience for me. I was sixteen years old and a junior when I started high school that fall. My school, at that time, was the largest in San Diego and the second largest in the state of California with thirty-two hundred students in grades ten, eleven, and twelve. Coming from a small school environment in Japan of two hundred students max where all my classmates were dependents of the U.S. military and almost everyone was comprised of mixed races, then transferring to this "city" they call a school in San Diego was an overwhelming culture shock. Although the school was integrated for purposes of racial equality, it was heavily divided socially into distinct races of White, Black, Hispanic, Samoan, and everyone else, and I was not accepted in any of these groups. I was already feeling very frightened and alone because my older sister Sachi had graduated and started school at a local college. So, in addition to being an outsider and feeling different from everyone else, I missed my sister and the blanket of sisterly love and protection she always provided. There were a few friends who were loners like me who gave me a sense of belonging especially during rowdy and segregated lunch periods. We usually brought lunch and ate outside in the courtyard under a tree. I somehow got through my junior and senior years at the same school with less than raving reviews from me, and graduated in June 1978 with eleven hundred fellow seniors, most of whom I never even met.

LIFE AS AN ADULT

As an adult, I held several jobs before landing the one I eventually retired from in 2009 at San Diego Superior Court as a Courtroom Clerk. Life at the Courts was interesting, exciting, and for the most part never a dull moment. Over the course of twenty years, I made acquaintances with countless wonderful people, many of them lawyers and judges, and several have become lifelong friends.

My home life with my husband of ten years was great until his life abruptly ended in 2008. Ron "Big Dawg" Billups, was a compassionate man who loved hard, worked hard, and played hard. He was Chicago-bred and brought that Midwest personality with him to California.

My parents passed away soon after the loss of my husband Ron - my mother in 2008 and my father in

2010. I am not alone; I have four wonderful children - three sons, Ronnie, Mario, and Ronald, a daughter, Miki and blessed with eight fantastic grandchildren - six boys and two girls.

HOT FLASH IS A SYMPTOM

After having such a wonderful childhood and a blessed life, my first hot flash was a sobering reality check. I felt like I had been doused with water. No! I wish I had been doused with water. How could life be so good and then go so wrong with these hot flashes?! What are they again…and where do they come from? Why am I getting them? Does everyone get them? Why? Does anyone know? These are some of the questions that were running through my mind when I had my first *real* hot flash, and what will be addressed in this chapter.

Before I delve into the topic of what hot flashes are, let me point out that "hot flashes" are just one of many symptoms of menopause, which brings us to the question - *what is menopause?* We should answer that question first since **hot flashes** are the by-product of menopause.

In the meantime and for your consideration, menopause symptoms include, but are not limited to the following:

- Hot flashes
- Fatigue
- Concentration & memory problems
- Headaches
- Bladder problems
- Breast tenderness
- Hair, nail & tooth problems

- Night sweats
- Insomnia
- Mood swings
- Vaginal dryness & itching
- Skin changes
- Bloating & gas
- Heavy or irregular bleeding

For the purpose of my book, however, I will primarily be addressing the hot flash symptom as it relates to menopause. Not because it tops the list as the most common of all menopause symptoms, but because it tops *my* list as the most distressing and disturbing.

WHAT IS MENOPAUSE?

When we hear the word "menopause" we tend to associate this term with older women, like our mothers, and something that's distant, detached, and far removed from us. However, menopause is something that occurs naturally in every woman's life and as women can't escape from. So, what do we do when it comes? The only thing we can do is embrace this new chapter, face it head-on and be well-equipped to endure. With menopause comes a certain stigma.

However, we do not have to treat it like a disease. We can take the time to learn more, and accept it as a part of life. Yes, menopause happens as we age. However, we are never too young to at least know something about it. So, stick around and enjoy the show, as they say.

The actual word "menopause" comes from the combined Greek root words of *meno* (month) and *pausis* (pause, cessation). It literally means a time in a woman's life when her *monthly* cycle *pauses* or ceases. To further complicate things, "menopause" has several different, yet similar, *terms* associated with the actual word "menopause", which is commonly known as "The Three Stages of Menopause" described here:

1) Peri-menopause - refers to the time before the end of a woman's monthly cycle

2) Menopause - refers to the time when a woman has gone twelve consecutive months without a monthly cycle

3) Post menopause - refers to the time after menopause

So, once a woman reaches that first stage, the next two are sure to follow. Age and the longevity of each stage vary with every woman. There's no measuring stick for this one. We can certainly glean from other women's experiences, but it's our own race to run when our time comes.

Think of going through menopause as puberty in reverse. During puberty *"hormones are gearing up for the reproductive years"* and during menopause the *"body is now turning them off."*

Let me clue you in to another word for menopause - *climacteric*. The dictionary definition for it is *"a major turning point or critical stage."* A more relevant definition is *"the years of symptoms that occur from the onset of ovarian decline to the time after menopause when symptoms stop."*

Now that we've been somewhat educated on the meaning of some of these menopausal buzz words, let's move on to this thing called "hot flash."

WHAT ARE HOT FLASHES?

Wikipedia defines "hot flashes" as follows:

> *"Hot flashes (also known as hot flushes) are a form of **flushing** due to reduced levels of **estradiol**. Hot flashes are a symptom which may have several other causes, but which is often caused by the changing **hormone** levels that are characteristic of **menopause**. They are typically experienced as a feeling of intense heat with sweating and rapid heartbeat, and may typically last from two to thirty minutes for each occurrence."*

My own personal definition of a hot flash is an unbelievable, uncontrollable, spontaneous inner combustion that manifests itself in the form of heat, sweat, pounding head and chest, dizziness, and temporary insanity. Get ready ladies - we may be in for a rough ride!

WHERE DO THEY COME FROM?

Simply put, *"a hot flash occurs because the brain decides your body is overheated."* Among other things, the temperature regulating system of a woman's body changes during menopause causing turmoil in the sweat glands and brain chemistry. For example, while the body's thermostat is struggling to reset itself during a fluctuation in body temperature caused by these sweat glands not working like they are supposed to, and brain chemistry affecting the hypothalamus or temperature control center, the body overcompensates causing a hot flash. That was the simple explanation.

The scientific term "vasomotor instability", often used to describe hot flashes, occurs when a decrease in estrogen levels cause blood vessel muscles to become less stable. What causes a decrease in estrogen levels? Primarily **age** - the body aging and going into menopause. Estrogen is a hormone produced by the ovaries along with the hormone progesterone. The pituitary gland in our brains produces a hormone called

Follicle Stimulating Hormone (FSH), which stimulates the production of estrogen. It has been thought that an increased level of this FSH may have something to do with the initiation of a hot flash. After all, it is a known medical fact that noticeable changes in FSH levels come with menopause and seem to be a direct result of the ovaries shrinking, leading to decreased levels of estrogen. I hope I didn't lose anyone there. I almost lost myself. It's all so relative, but very confusing.

DOES EVERYONE GET THEM?

The answer is a resounding "no" according to medical sources across the board. Actually only about seventy-five percent of menopausal women will experience hot flashes. That's good news for the remaining twenty-five percent of the female menopausal population. Congratulations sisters and please enjoy your freedom from these hot flashes as the rest of us take one for the team. I am so happy for you and envious at the same time. I cannot wait for the day when I can wear regular clothes again. You'll learn more about that in Chapter Five!

WHY SOME AND NOT OTHERS?

This a big question. Why do some women get hot flashes and others don't? I believe the answer lies somewhere deep within the physiological makeup and chemistry of each individual woman. The short of it? It's complex. It primarily depends on those estrogen and FSH levels and how they are being produced in the body until they are no longer present.

Remember fifth grade health education class where we had to learn about male and female reproductive systems? Well, allow me to refresh your memory. The rise and fall of estrogen and progesterone levels during a woman's ovulation period is a direct result of whether or not an egg was fertilized and therefore has everything to do with a woman either becoming pregnant or having a monthly cycle. So, when a woman is in menopause, her body starts to produce less estrogen and progesterone, which causes the monthly cycle to become less regular to the point where it sooner or later stops.

Some experts believe that women who may have experienced severe symptoms during their puberty years may also have a trying menopause. On the other hand, those who had an easy go of their adolescent years may experience menopause with no hardship. Who knows? The two may go hand in hand. To use myself as an example, severe symptoms were normal for me during puberty. My monthly cycle started at age twelve and every month I experienced terrible symptoms like heavy bleeding, excruciating cramps, and annoying headaches. It wasn't until the birth of my first child that these symptoms lessened. Now that

I am menopausal, severe hot flash symptoms occur. So, there may be some truth to that theory.

I can go on and on boring you with endless reasons why doctors, researchers, and medical science have no concrete answers to this valid yet mind-boggling question, *"Why do some women get them (hot flashes) and others don't?"* It has become increasingly obvious to me that there are probably no real answers that predict whether a woman will be prone to having hot flashes or not. Simple as that. In my opinion, I feel ongoing research has produced nothing new on this subject - nada, nil, zilch, zero - not because of lack of interest or effort, but because of the complex nature of the human body. As a doctor once said, *"the essence of the peri-menopause is its variability, and that is what makes it so hard to study."*

So, in the unscientific world, some might say it's just the luck of the draw not to have hot flashes. While others may think they are cursed for having them. But neither is the case. A medical expert put it this way,

> *"...if you have hot flashes and your best friend doesn't, don't think, even for one minute, that she is in any way 'better' than you. It's your body chemistry, not your mind."*

I say amen to that, and consider yourself blessed if you never had to or have to experience them! For those of us who do, well, let's go through it with our dignity intact and our heads held high. We, too, are blessed. Our road may have a few more bumps in it than the others, but we can look forward to smoother sailing down the road!

CULTURAL DIVERSITY

Chotto matte! That means "wait a minute!" in Japanese. Let me share just one more thing before closing this chapter - something I learned about *cultural differences* when it comes to women and menopause. This is fascinating, promise! I never thought women in other cultures experience menopause, too. But why wouldn't they? We are all women no matter where we are from or where we live.

Like anything else, cultural differences in menopausal women can be identified through a well-monitored reporting system based on many factors. In the case of menopausal women worldwide, the difference in diet, exercise and language can affect the outcome of these reports. For instance, did you know that there is no exact translation for the word "hot flash" in the Japanese language? It's described more like "blushing." Because of this slight difference and language barrier, there is a much lower reported incidence of hot flashes in Japanese women. Pretty amazing, huh? That's just one interesting fact about one culture.

For those of you who would like to learn more about cultural differences in menopausal women, there is a worldwide organization called the *"International Menopause Society"* *(IMS)* that you may wish to consider. Their website (www.imsociety.org) is loaded with good information about menopausal women from all over the world (under the heading *"Menopause Perspectives"*). It may be worth your while to also check out the *"North American Menopause Society"* *(NAMS)*. Their website is www.menopause.org.

This chapter has a lot of information to digest because it was a lot for me to sift through. I do hope you have a clearer understanding of what hot flashes are, where they come from, who can get them, how long they last, and how it's all a part of the "change of life" we call menopause. I know I do.

CHAPTER 2

UNCOVERING THE HEAT

I have noticed that most women don't share their hot flash experiences with anyone except maybe their doctor. Why is that? First of all, most women don't like to bother anyone with their health issues. Am I right? Second, it's too embarrassing to talk about. Who wants to talk about sweat let alone our own sweat? Third, hot flashes generally don't last long enough to give them any merit for discussion. My average hot flash (yes I timed them) lasts 60 seconds or less. That's just enough time for people around you to not really notice unless you point it out to them. If they do notice, they may think you're just naturally hot or it's something not out of the ordinary. So they ignore you. Women, in general, do not like bringing undue negative attention to themselves, especially during a hot flash. I'd rather people didn't notice. I just subtly fan myself and have learned to carry a small towel, handkerchief, or paper towel on me at all times.

Historically, women have been known to not talk about certain topics publicly like menopause and menstruation. I found in my research that women and menopause in the World War II generation differ considerably from women today both socially as well as politically. It was a different time for our ancestral sisters back then. Women were, for the most part, silent and they certainly did not have the political backing to support their female issues. That's why I believe people, particularly in my generation, never knew our grandmothers even went through menopause nor did we hear our own mothers talk about it, let alone have discussions with us - the children. So, it feels as though we're on our own, shockingly, even in this day and age. These may be considered modern times, and time has definitely brought about change when it comes to the discussion of female issues, but I don't hear women in my age group openly talking about menopause. Younger women in their forties might be having a chat or two about it, or maybe I'm just hanging out with the wrong crowd - no offense to anyone. Although broaching the subject of menopause is definitely more socially accepted among women today, I still don't think it's a totally comfortable topic that's brought up casually in everyday conversations.

Even behind closed doors in the doctor's office, it's not really discussed in great detail. No disrespect to doctors, but we as women are often told that it's the "change of life," expect it, take estrogen, and it will go away eventually. We accept that and go out into the real world hot flashing all over the place often making everyone around us as miserable as we are.

Pump the brakes ladies! We don't have to put ourselves in a box on a shelf to hide from the rest of the world. We shouldn't place ourselves in isolation because our condition isn't contained. We shouldn't have to feel ashamed of this natural occurrence in our body just because everyone else around us has no clue of what we're going through. Well, I say here's our chance to be ourselves and tell the world! Let's tackle this problem together, shall we? Are you game?

Let me take you back to grade school where we learned the "who, what, where, when, and why" in English class. We are going to apply that technique to this chapter of uncovering the heat. We know the "who" is us, the "what" are the hot flashes, the "where" is anywhere, and the "when" is whenever. The "why" is the question we want to answer in this chapter as it relates to *why* we, as women, are so reluctant or afraid to openly talk about our hot flashes. Then we can focus on the "how." Now, let's go and uncover this heat!

MY FIRST HOT FLASH

When I experienced my first hot flash, yes, I was embarrassed. But *why* is that? Let's explore the psychological implications of my embarrassment. I can identify four things that led to my embarrassment - pride, awareness, exposure, self-consciousness. First, let's begin with *"pride"*, which is *conceit* or *justifiable self-respect*. I'm leading off with *pride* because it is the root of many issues concerning emotions and feelings including embarrassment. When we feel embarrassed, it's often because our *"pride"* is affected in some way - usually through hurt or humiliation. So, *"pride"* is number one. Next, we have *"awareness"*, which means *having perception or knowledge*. What made me feel embarrassed at the moment of my first hot flash was *awareness*. I suddenly became *"aware"* of something new and foreign, and felt *embarrassed* because something different and unfamiliar was going on in my body that was uncontrollable, and feared everyone could see but me. It's like having food stuck between your teeth or an unsightly pimple on your face, toilet paper stuck to the bottom of your shoe, your blouse open more than you intended, your shirt mis-buttoned or your fly open. Everyone around you can see these things except you. The strange looks, stares, giggles, sneers, smiles received, or maybe that kind someone finally pointing it out makes you *aware* of the source of all the undue attention. So, *"awareness"* is number two.

After becoming *aware*, your eyes are opened to a situation that is now *"exposed"* or *caused to be open to view*. "Exposed" is number three. I was now out there for the whole world to witness me having a hot flash

- whatever that may look like. It doesn't matter how it appears, people can still see me. Now comes all the questions of insecurity - what do I look like at this very moment? Can they see the sweat beads running down my face and neck? Because it sure feels like Niagara Falls rushing down my back. Am I turning colors? Because I am feeling awfully hot. Do I look like I'm about to pass out? Because I feel really light-headed. Is my mouth gaped wide open? Because I'm in total shock right now. Are there any body fluids coming out of me that I should know about? Because I'm numb and I can't feel a thing right now. A hundred and one similar questions ran through my mind all at once and I didn't have an answer for any of them. I wanted to get up and run just like the thoughts that were running through my mind, but my bottom felt glued to my seat. *Why* did I suddenly have the urge to run away? Because I was now *"self-conscious"* or *uncomfortably conscious of myself as an object of observation by others*. This is number four - *"self-conscious."* I was *self-conscious* of what I might be looking like to other people and because I couldn't see at that moment. A glimpse might make me feel a little better.

True story: I knew a young lady once who would prop a small mirror up against something on the table in front of her whenever she ate in public. When I asked her why, she simply replied, so she could see if any food stuck in her teeth or if something was on her face before anyone else could to avoid being embarrassed. At the time this seemed like overkill, but now I sure wish I had a mirror at the moment of my first hot flash!

To sum it all up, the embarrassment caused by the sudden onset of my hot flash affected my *pride* because I became *aware* I'd been *exposed* to everyone around me, making me feel very *self-conscious*. So, there you have it - the "why" according to me and my first hot flash experience. This may be why women are so reluctant or afraid to openly talk about their hot flashes. In one word, it's *embarrassing!*

WHAT DO I DO?

Now that I was feeling all of these things, what do I do with them or about them? Quick! Run! Hide! Take cover and never come out! That's how I felt, but that's not what we have to resort to. We have the option of taking our embarrassing hot flash moments in stride and not letting it undermine us or who we are. We can still strut our stuff and display ourselves like the peacocks we are. That's right! To women everywhere, let the world see us in all of our splendor. We are beautiful! Speaking of peacocks, let me share with you an interesting fact about these colorful creatures that I learned from a very fascinating article I read! Here's the link to the article, and I also included the excerpt about the peacocks for you below:

http://www.oprah.com/inspiration/The-Unexpected-Route-to-a-Spiritual-Miracle

"The Unexpected Route to a Spiritual Miracle"
By Marianne Williamson
(The author of Tears to Triumph)

"In order to create their beautiful plumage, peacocks sometimes eat thorns. Hard, pointed, razorlike objects are processed in their abdomens and then contribute to feathers with colors and shapes unmatched throughout nature for their extraordinary beauty. So it is with us.

Often, that which is the hardest to digest, to process, to integrate into our life experiences is what ultimately transforms us in a positive way. We become who we are meant to be sometimes by having to eat some hard-edged, bitter thorns of human experience."

Isn't that amazing? Although the author is obviously not talking about hot flashes, I was inspired by her comparison of the peacocks' transformation to our own human experiences.

Like the author, Marianne Williamson, there are many, many, many books, articles, and blogs out there where people share their own human experiences about a variety of subjects. And that brings us to the "how." Why not share our experiences about the forbidden or less talked about subject - *women and hot flashes*? There are some good books out there written on the subject by medical doctors and experts, but they center more around the clinical aspect of hot flashes. I believe there should be more books written and published from a woman's perspective about their own personal hot flash experiences. Even though we may not like *talking* about it, I think most women wouldn't mind *learning* more, and that can happen through reading. It's always very comforting to me to read about something I'm already going through. In addition to it being informative, it can be relatable, affirming, reassuring, and self-validating to know you are not experiencing something by yourself and that you share common ground with someone even outside your circle of family and friends. Most women like to read, and besides reading gives us the quiet time we so often need but don't always have because of our busy and hectic schedules. So, my lady warriors, let's rise to the occasion. Think about it…and share. How? Well, in your own words, of course, and in your own way - whether it's one-on-one with a girlfriend, in a group setting, over the phone, written text, email, video, social media, blogs, or the world wide web. It's your soap box and the world is your oyster!

As *sharing* goes, my immediate family and closest friends have seen my hot flash moments. Some may comment, but don't usually take it any further by elaborating. I find this especially true for males and women who have never had a hot flash, because they don't know what to say. How can they speak on something they know nothing about?

For instance, when I mentioned to my oldest son, Ronnie, that I was writing this book about hot flashes, his mind went back to when his grandmother was having hot flashes. It didn't dawn on him back then, of course, because he was just a child. But looking back now as an adult, it all started to make sense to him. He even recalled something I had forgotten about - his grandmother always had a towel wrapped around her neck. *And she did!* It wasn't just any towel. It was a Japanese towel. What's so special about that? Well, the Japanese wash cloth is this extra long towel that is used to scrub their backs in an easy side-to-side motion. This towel is long, but not thick. It became the perfect towel for my mother to hang around her neck without it being cumbersome. So, having this conversation with my son opened up his understanding about women and hot flashes. Although he and my other children have witnessed me, their own mother, having hot flashes, they never really pursued it further to learn more. This is not a reprimand - it's just a fact of life, something people don't really talk about. A stigma.

So, I have learned to make light of it and offer a simple explanation to my family and friends as to why

I'm so hot all the time, phrasing it in a way that isn't awkward and they actually get it. This also opens the door for them to inquire further. If they ask a question, I give them an honest answer and like to think that when they ask questions they're either curious, concerned, or both. If you see your family and circle of friends regularly, they get to know you and your hot flashes and will accept them as part of your makeup for the time being or they will ask how you're doing with them. Either way, it's a live conversation and one that's being *shared*.

There are countless people on this earth who do not share their true feelings. I was one of them, but what I discovered is, when I kept things to myself, my thoughts and feelings, good and "not so good", had nowhere to go but to internalize within me. So, eventually the thoughts and feelings that were "not so good" festered and grew in very harmful ways until it became toxic like poison - simply because of not sharing them with others. I was in a relationship that wasn't emotionally healthy, and slowly over a span of time became distant and isolated from the rest of the world including my family. I didn't really notice until awaking one day feeling unfulfilled. My life only *existed* here on earth, I wasn't really *living*, just taking up space and burning a hole through it. I needed help. After finally taking an honest look at my situation, I became aware of not surrounding myself with positive people. My friends at that time started dropping off one by one until there were none. So, without friends meant I wasn't sharing my fears and concerns with trustworthy people or those who could help me. Where was I and what was I doing with my life? Sixty years of age was now closer than fifty, and that became an eye opener for me. I could not go on wasting any more time. What was I waiting for? Seventy? I almost waited too late and it was time to make a move.

By some miracle during that time, a dear friend called out of the blue to check on me. They asked enough of the right questions to know something was very wrong with me and my situation. From there, the ability to *share* my circumstance with someone who had a positive energy flow helped me climb out of my hole of despair and take my life back. Not *sharing* one's thoughts can be deadly serious. No one should ever have to feel like they're alone or go through anything by themselves - especially a difficult or seemingly hopeless situation.

Yes, I may have shared a little more than you expected, but that part of me is a part of this book. I have learned that by not *sharing* experiences - good or not so good - can be damaging and even dangerous. On the flip side, it may even be considered selfish to have information that can help someone in a positive way and you withhold it by not *sharing*. So, you see, I am not only happy, but obligated to share with you my story. My friend, be encouraged, take heart and gather up the courage to *share* your story with someone who may need to hear it. You never know whose life you may touch, help climb out of the dark pit of despair or even save. If you are that one in the hole, please reach out today and find the "strength and courage", as my sister Sachi would say, to seek help from the right person or persons so you can start living your life again - happy and fulfilled. That hole is dark and lonely and it wasn't made for you. Please come and join the rest of us on the sunny side of life!

CHAPTER 3

HE DOESN'T GET IT

From a woman's perspective a man doesn't get hot flashes just like he doesn't get childbirth or our monthly cycle thing, or why we shop so much or pretty much anything involving women where men have to think. Am I being hard on men? No. That's just the way they're wired. Just like we women are wired in our own unique way. When it comes to certain "female" topics men tend to shy away from talking about them. It makes them uncomfortable and squeamish. They twist and squirm until they can't hide it any more. Then they scratch their head and find an excuse to walk away or, in some cases, run. (You can run, but you can't hide!) Let me share with you something my husband once told me that one of his friends said to him about women and their monthly cycle. Warning! It's a bit graphic. So, I'm apologizing in advance. This friend said he doesn't trust anyone who bleeds for 3-4 days straight every month and doesn't die. What kind of a thing is that to say! Do all men feel this way? I mean it's funny, but it's not funny. That kind of comment just makes women want to cock their head to the side and give men that look. You know the look!

That's why men aren't equipped to have conversations like this with women about women and their hot little "oven" or their "childbearing factory." Truth be told, men are only interested when it becomes the "pleasure factory." On the real though, men's opinions about women are all over the place - they can go from one end of the spectrum to the other.

So, for that reason, I decided to include a chapter just for men. Yay! Or should I say hoo-rah! I want men to feel comfortable when their wife or partner is going through this "change of life" thing. I want you men to feel confident and be able to pick up on some of the warning signs that come with this phase in a woman's life. I want to help men help themselves so they can help their wives and keep their marriage or relationship intact. This can be a stressful time for women, and stress can add to the intensity of the hot flashes. No one wants that, trust me!

WOMEN ARE CRAZY! BUT YA GOTTA LOVE 'EM!

Men, you say you don't know what to do. Well, good news, you don't have to do *anything*. Don't think in terms of *chores*. Just pay attention, open your ears, and hear what your wife is saying to you. I know it's hard sometimes because we take forever explaining stuff and we tend to speak in riddles or circles and expect you to understand exactly what we're saying. Yes, we can be downright unreasonable. So much so that it makes men want to throw their hands up in the air in exasperation and as a sign of giving up. Admit it, women, we drive them a little crazy in more ways than one sometimes. Take, for example, the movie *"White Men Can't Jump"* where the main character Billy throws a glass of water on his live-in girlfriend Gloria because she said one thing and meant another and expected him to know what she was talking about from some magazine article she read. Really??? I probably would have done the same thing if I were a guy. Sorry, fellow female cohorts, but I have to admit we are like that at times and it's not always fair to our male counterparts. But men, we women, for the most part, just want to vent. You don't even have to process what we're saying (because we'll repeat it for you if you ask us to!). Listen men, we don't want you to *fix* it. We just want you to *listen* to us and actually *hear* the words that we are saying. (Vent! Vent!! Vent!!!) It takes time and patience to listen to us - something you men don't have if it doesn't involve a ball being lobbed across a field or court somewhere. But try to give your woman your undivided attention when she's feeling a certain way.

And women - hear me when I say this - PLEASE try to give your man some consideration when he's watching TV or hanging out with the guys. Choose the right time and place where you both can give each other the quiet, uninterrupted time that you deserve. This is important. You will be surprised just how a few minutes of talking to each other in an open and honest dialogue can bring many years of happiness. That's all I'll say about that. I'm done lecturing. Oh, one last thing, a word from the wise - my Dad - he would always say to me and my husband, "Take care of each other." It's a simple statement, but it's strong and profound.

So, how does a male react to a woman's hot flash? Men, hello, admit it. If a woman was having a hot flash, would you even know she was having a hot flash, and should you even be looking? Are you looking because your damsel-in-distress signal just kicked in and you want to help? Or did your male hormones pick up a hot, sweaty woman on its radar? Well, that's just fine and dandy. Let me help you out. If she's not your woman, ignore her unless she faints. Then call for help. If she is your woman, you'll be loved so much more if you just ask her nicely if there's anything you can do for her. Simple as that! If there is, she'll tell you, and then do it with a smile! If this works, you can thank me by sharing it with all your male friends. If this doesn't work, then just leave her alone until you can figure something else out.

Let me help you out again. It helps to know little things about your woman - like her favorite drink (doesn't have to be alcohol) in her favorite cup, her favorite chair, her favorite blanket or pillow, her favorite room in the house, her favorite book or magazine, her favorite food or snack, her favorite movie or TV show, her favorite color, and the list goes on. Once you know these things, you are better equipped to serve her. Women are usually impressed when their man knows the little things that they like, their dislikes, and the idiosyncrasies about them. (Not to insult your intelligence, but an idiosyncrasy is a *"funny quirk or habit that makes a person different."* Don't worry - I admit I didn't know how to spell it.)

Take another movie, for example, *"Me Before You,"* where the main character Louisa Clarke squeals for joy and runs out of the room when William, the man she was hired to caretake, gives her as a birthday gift a pair of black and yellow striped tights that she loved since childhood. Seconds before that, Louisa's boyfriend gave her a specially made silver heart-shaped pendant necklace with his name "Patrick" in the middle of the heart to which she uttered a stiff "thank you." Do you see the difference? One gift was thoughtful and the other was self-serving. The striped tights were simple and probably inexpensive, but according to the movie they were also very hard to find. So, the thoughtfulness came from William when: 1) he paid attention to

Louisa when she first told him her childhood story about wearing the tights everyday until she outgrew them physically and couldn't find them anywhere in her now adult size, and 2) he took the time to find them and then gave them to her as a gift. Women are sentimental creatures and very emotional, thus the two very different reactions from Louisa to her gifts. Now, don't get me wrong. Women love jewelry, cars, houses, and vacations to exotic places as gifts too, so don't think you can get away with giving us a small thoughtful gift for every occasion. See how we are, men? Hard to please and hard to figure out. But seriously, women love gifts period - just choose the right one for the right occasion. On an everyday level, like hot flashes, women love the little things that let them know you listen and you care. Now that's BIG, and hey, you don't have to rub it in their face and take credit for it with a lot of big talk. Just smile and enjoy the moment! You'll get your chance to gloat when she settles down and asks you how you knew. (Here's a secret - William's response to Louisa's question in the movie was, "It's a secret.")

And take your time when catering to her. Don't make her feel like she's second fiddle to anything - the TV, your games, your hobbies, your car, your motorcycle, your Mom, your friends, or your kids. If you make her first fiddle, you will be treated like a king. Then you can go play with your other fiddles. And that doesn't mean other women - watch yourself!

WHADDYA DO?

Am I still talking about hot flashes? You betcha! Hot flashes are HOOOOT - number one! They're also annoying, debilitating, and tiresome - number two. So, patience is what's needed here. This can go on for days, weeks, months, or even years! Each hot flash can last from a minute or two or, in severe cases, up to thirty minutes or more. The intensity can vary, too, from a mild, prissy fan-waving hot to "get me a friggin' freezer I can sit in!" hot. Let me rephrase that for you. That would be like you "shooting-a-few-basketball-hoops-by-yourself" hot, to "playing-a-full-court-game-with-the-guys" hot. Feel me? Yep.

So, whaddya do? Divorce her? No! Leave her? No! Well, maybe for a few hours. Remember, this is a temporary condition. I know I said years, but in many cases it may last a year or less. But if you turn out to be one of the "lucky" ones who has to deal with it for a few years or more, please get some help! No, really. Get to know your woman and what makes her tick. If you haven't already taken the time to do this, now would be a good time. Don't be shy - remember this is new for her, too. While she's trying to figure it out, you be right there in the wings with her. Take notes if you have to - no shame in that. You know how you guys easily forget stuff. I'd like to think it's not on purpose, but jot it down!

READ THE FLASHING SIGNS

Just to be fair to you men, let me level the playing field a bit and give you a few good inside tips you need to know about women. I can't send you out there clueless! Don't worry, ladies, I won't give away all of our secrets - just a few to get some help from our well-intended hunks.

So, what can you men *really* do for your hot flashing woman? Leave her to her own devices and she'll be fine. Because what you don't want to do is *over* do it. I know this sounds like a contradiction to what's been said so far when it comes to catering to your woman, but it's a pretty thin line between making a woman feel special and getting on her last nerve. You have to be able to read the signs guys - the flashing signs, the hot flashing signs. Sometimes they're loud and clear and other times they are silent and almost non-existent. Learn your woman. Know ahead of time what it takes to please her and what's going to set her off. You almost have to be psychic to predict her reactions.

As a bonus, I'm going to help you out by first giving you a crash course on women, not just the hot flashing ones. So, listen up - you don't want to miss this.

Aside from the obvious in-your-face confrontations, some of the most misunderstood signs that a woman is annoyed are her facial expressions, her body language, the silent treatment, and tears. You don't want to misinterpret or ignore any of these signs because they will lead to a slammed door or two in your face, flying objects in your direction, screaming or yelling, more tears or an old fashioned conniption fit. Need some examples? Here are a few signs to watch for when a woman is annoyed:

FACIAL EXPRESSIONS

The Lips

- When a woman's lips are pursed together in a thin straight line, she is annoyed. How can you tell? Because she's not talking and women love to talk.
- If there's a twist on those tight lips, it's pretty bad.
- If she has an eyebrow raised on top of that, brace yourself for a tongue lashing sooner or later.
- When a woman pouts, it's because she didn't get her way. Think of something quick or you'll get the silent treatment. Or even worse, a huge credit card bill.

The Eyes

- If she rolls her eyes at you, she's sick and tired of whatever it is you're doing or saying. Best thing to do is to stop doing it.

- If she avoids looking at you altogether, you've really pissed her off. So, figure it out and apologize to her.
- If her eyes are closed and her eyebrows are knit closely together, she's not hearing you. So, just stop talking until she's ready to hear you.
- When she's looking at you with both eyebrows raised and cranes her neck like E.T., she's waiting for an answer from you. So, don't blow it by saying something dumb or stupid.

BODY LANGUAGE

Folded arms

- She is cross with you
- She's not happy about something
- She's waiting for you make something right

Hands on hips

- She's wants something done and is waiting for you to get off you tush (tapping foot)
- She's assessing what you've done and trying to decide if she likes or not (head cocked to one side)

Turns her back to you

- She's upset about something you did or said
- She *doesn't* want to hear what you have to say

Tilts her head up to the sky with her nose in the air

- She's upset about something you did or said
- She's *waiting* to hear what you have to say

SILENT TREATMENT

She walks away, leaves the room, leaves the house

- Like turning her back to you, she's upset about something you did or said
- She's protesting something - like being on strike
- She will stay silent for as long as she feels necessary

Snatches her hand or body away from you

- She's mad and hurt about something you did or said
- She doesn't want to talk about it right now
- She needs time to stew about it

Avoids eye contact

- Again, she's in protest - on strike
- She wants you to feel her pain
- She's not going to speak until:
  - The wrong is made right
  - She decides it's not worth it by being silent
  - Being silent is costing her the freedom to talk

TEARS

Tears are a very hard thing for men and women to deal with. Contrary to popular belief, women don't generally like to cry. I know that we sometimes use it to our benefit to get our way with men - and women sometimes, believe it or not. When women are reduced to crying, it's usually because a button deep down inside of our emotional psyche has been pushed causing the dam to break and the waterworks to flow, and in some cases, overflow. Once that first tear falls, it's impossible to reverse it. Women feel that if we start crying, we may as well let it all hang out. Because if you witnessed the first tear roll, it's over. There's no taking it back. Our cool composure has been blown and there's nothing left to hide.

Now, men, there's crying and then there's uncontrollable crying. This is something you want to avoid at all costs because the outcome can be very unpredictable. Assuming that your woman is sincerely crying about something you did to upset her, sobbing uncontrollably means it has overtaken her entire being. She has resorted to the only thing left to do when there are no more words to make her feel better. Depending on the situation, there may be no coming back from this one. But if you wish to try, I suggest trying to console her by gently putting your arm - just one arm - around her. If she doesn't resist, try both arms in a loose, but comforting hug. If she sobs even harder, then and only then, you can hold her closer and tighter. Don't say anything for a few minutes. Remember what I said about women being emotional creatures. Hugging is a very comforting and emotional thing for us. If you start talking, she may start talking and this may upset her all over again to the point of breaking away from your hug and being madder than she was in the first place.

I know I went a little deep with that, but it's important to know and understand these things. It will be beneficial to you in the long run.

READ THE HOT FLASHING SIGNS

So, now that you've been educated on reading the signs of an annoyed woman, let's get back to reading the signs of your hot flashing woman. Any or all of the following can happen during a hot flash:

- Her forehead gets sweaty and she looks a little dazed
- She stops doing a task to sit down
- She leans back and closes her eyes (jaws clenched)
- She loses focus while you're talking to her (blank stare)
- Her chest, neck, or upper arms turn a blotchy red
- She suddenly starts to fan herself
- She turns on the A/C or fan

Here are a few simple, on-target, no fuss, instant relief things you can do for her while she's having a hot flash:

- Ask her in a light tone, *"Can I get you something from the fridge, _____?"* (You fill in the blank with "babe, dear, honey" etc.) And don't assume you know what she needs or wants. Let her tell you.
- Gently place a cool damp cloth *in her hands* - don't just drop it in her lap or on her head.
- Quietly turn on the fan or A/C even if it's just for a few minutes.

The key here is to just act natural and be casual. Don't bring attention to it. No big fanfare. She just wants to cool off.

Let me tell you a cute little story about one of my grandsons, Brayden, who is five years old. During one of my recent visits, I had a hot flash. I was in Brayden's room watching him play his favorite video game when I suddenly got hot and mumbled to myself, "It's *hot* in here." I didn't mean for him to hear me and I intended to get up and turn on the ceiling fan myself. Without missing a beat, Brayden paused his game, jumped off the bed, and turned on the ceiling fan. Simple as that. This really impressed me for several reasons: 1) the fact that he even heard me at all because he was so focused on his game; 2) he saw a problem and knew how to solve it; 3) he didn't hesitate, but took immediate action; and 4) he cared enough about his grandma to want to make her feel comfortable (just like his older brother Jalen, who at the age of four, was a great source of comfort to me when I lost my husband in 2008). What Brayden did for me took less than five seconds, and that, guys, deserves a high five!

So, if a five-year old boy can figure out what to do for his grandma who he sees once or twice a year, certainly a man should know what to do for the wife he's been living with for many years to make her feel comfortable.

Do you get it now? Have I made it crystal clear? You got this, man! You can do it. I have faith in you!

GET A ROOM!

Now make room for the bedroom! Yes, the sanctuary, the cave, the haven, heaven, the baby-making room, the place where all things happen that are only between you and her. Did I put too much on it? Well, whatever you call it, the bedroom may become a place where the two of you just *sleep* together for awhile. When a woman is hot flashing through the night, SHE DOES NOT WANT TO BE BOTHERED WITH YOU! Let me say that again. When a woman is hot flashing through the night, SHE DOES NOT WANT TO BE BOTHERED WITH YOU! Don't be offended - it's not you! A hot flash, or in this case, a night sweat can become so hot even she doesn't want to be bothered with her own self - let alone YOU! So, don't get mad. Roll over and go back to sleep or take a cold shower. Sorry! I know that's like a kick in the pants, but you *do not* want to make love to a woman who is hot flashing - trust me - unless you want to get slapped or worse. You won't get any action though - I'll tell you that. It would be like humping a sack of flour or worse - not happening, hon'! So, get a room! Not a hotel room, silly. I mean another room in the house.

I wonder if that's why couples in my parent's generation started sleeping in different beds or had separate bedrooms in their older age. My parents eventually ended up in separate bedrooms with their own beds (twin beds at that!), their own TV's, and everything. It became a way of life for them. The same was true for my husband's parents. They, too, had separate bedrooms. I remember my husband asking his parents about it on one of our visits. My guess is he found it strange seeing it for the first time. I don't recall if he got an answer that satisfied his curiosity. The thought never crossed my mind to ask my parents. I just assumed my mother had the window open all the time and my father was always cold, and at their age, they were probably too old to well - you know.

Now, I'm not saying you should have separate beds or sleep in separate rooms, but it may not be a bad idea to have a spare bed or couch ready in another room or another part of the house for those occasional nights when it becomes unbearable for her to the point where she kicks you out of the bed. Better to leave the room than to leave the house, right? Don't allow giving her space to hurt your ego. She will appreciate you a lot more, and joy will come in the morning, amen?

I don't want to leave you without hope. So, here's my suggestion. Wanting to be intimate with your woman can be tricky, but don't give up! Just time the hot flashes and proceed accordingly. This requires planning and spontaneity. If nighttime doesn't do it for you, perhaps a morning quickie or an afternoon delight. Just make sure it's consensual - know what I mean?

WOMEN ARE NOT IGUANAS

Men, I know you don't want to hear this, but please be thankful you don't have hot flashes. Be glad you're not the hot one in this book! For me, it's been one of the toughest things I've had to endure, perhaps because they're ongoing. It wouldn't be so bad if it happened only once or twice, like my friend Martha who literally only had *one hot flash* during her menopause experience! If this were the case, we would not even be having this conversation right now.

Hot flashes are real and they affect a great number of women. Very few of us are fortunate enough to escape this hotbox experience. Hot flashes are inconvenient and seem to come at the most inopportune times, but when you want one to come because it's cold outside - they don't. Funny how that works.

Once, a friend of mine was shocked because I was cold at an outdoor evening event. He said, "But you're always hot." I rolled my eyes and said, "No, I'm always cold by nature. The hot flashes make me hot and only when I'm having one." That's true. Before my hot flashes, I was someone who was always cold. I even kept a small heater and poncho at my desk at work. Nowadays, I am hot a lot, but only when I'm hot flashing. When I'm not hot flashing, I get cold when it's cold.

We women are not iguanas or those lizards with thick scaly skin that can adapt to any temperature. We feel the hot and cold just like everybody else. So, please don't make that comment my friend did if your wife decides to bring a wrap with her on a night outing. Just nod your head in acknowledgment, open her car door, and be on your way.

ALMOST DONE HERE

So, men, I hope this chapter was helpful to you. I hope that you are able to take some of these lessons and apply them to your relationships successfully and in a positive way.

You don't have to stop here. You are welcome to continue reading. In fact, there's more for you in the last chapter if you wanted to skip to the end of the book. Thanks for your attention.

CHAPTER 4

WHEN THE REAL ONE HITS

AT THE RESTAURANT

My hot flash journey began on January 6, 2011 with my first *real* hot flash - the mother of all hot flashes. Let me set the stage. My family and I just got seated at a restaurant and were looking at the menu when "it" came. I remember thinking, "What was THAT?!" I was wearing a silk chiffon blended top that literally stuck to the front and back of my clammy body when this tidal wave of unexpected heat invaded my body. It left as suddenly as it came leaving me dazed, stunned, and swimming in my own sweat. I felt far away and lost in a momentary lapse of consciousness. Coming back to my senses, I saw my dinner companions staring back at me with concern. Embarrassment was written all over my face. I looked around nervously hoping no one noticed and whispered, "I think I just had my first hot flash…" I didn't process it then, but I now recall my sister just nodding her head, eyebrows raised and without even looking at me she exhaled and softly said, "Wow!" My niece let out a youthful laugh, after seeing I was okay and didn't seem to think any more about it. But deep inside my thoughts, I could not believe my first real, genuine, legitimate, bonafide HOT FLASH had happened! My breath was literally taken away! I wasn't so shocked that it happened, because I knew it would occur one day. Flabbergasted best describes my mindset at the time because it happened while in the public view of so many people, and this wasn't just any old eating establishment. This was an upscale restaurant in a high-rise building in the heart of downtown during a peak dinner hour! How could I be hot flashing right now? This wasn't supposed to happen right here right now. It was supposed to happen late at night while I was asleep in bed. Why did I think that? Let me tell you why.

SATIN PAJAMAS

About ten years before my restaurant hot flash, an older sister of one of my dearest girlfriends shared with me her hot flash experience. I was at her house one day just visiting. She was a stay-at-home mom. Although it was well past mid-morning, she was dressed in her pajamas, which seemed a little odd at the time. In any case, I remember her wearing a beautiful shiny sky blue satin pair of pajamas - matching top and bottom, which looked gorgeous against her youthful-looking dark skin. She was about ten years older than me. I complimented her on her appearance and this was her response, *"Oh, I don't always look like this. I can't wear this to bed."* I did not understand her comment and after asking her why, she said it was because she sweats at night. She could see I was perplexed, so she continued to explain by saying, *"Oh, just wait till yours comes. You'll be sleeping at night and it will wake you up. You'll be sleeping good, too! But you'll get so hot! I'm talking hot, hot, hot! So hot I have to kick the covers off! Then I'm soaking wet from sweating so much, I have to change my clothes."* By this time my mouth was hanging open in disbelief and I finally let out a nervous laugh. I didn't know what to say and had no idea what she was talking about. Then she said it again, *"Just wait till yours comes. You'll know."*, and shaking her head, she added, *"Nothin' like it."* That's all she said. I didn't know what to make of that conversation and dismissed it, not really giving it any more thought.

BACK AT THE RESTAURANT

So, back at the restaurant, I couldn't get that hot flash out of my mind and remember thinking so many different thoughts I could hardly concentrate on the food in front of me. What was going on? What was I going to do? What's going to happen to me now? What do other women do when they get this? Oh my God, am I officially in menopause? I felt like I did when I first started my monthly cycle at the tender age of twelve. Knowing it was coming, but not knowing what to expect. This was devastating. My life was over. I'm old. I'm not young any more. I almost wanted my periods to come back. Whoa! That's how I felt on my first real hot flash.

What particularly stuck out as I started to think ahead a bit was, "I have to rethink my wardrobe. I'll never be able to wear silk, chiffon, rayon, or anything beautiful again! I'll be stuck wearing something old and ugly and I'll, for sure, have to wear an undershirt or something. What's that going to be like?" I remember wondering.

On the heels of that first real hot flash were many more hot flashes than I even care to count. Here's the break down of my hot flash journey in three parts - the *beginning*, *middle*, and *end*. I'll call the one before my real one hit *the beginning*. When the real one hit will be the *middle* and it's also where I am today. So, for me, the *end* of my hot flash journey is still to come - somewhere in the *near* future, I hope. Oh please, please, please!

BACK TO THE BEGINNING

Allow me to back up and start at the _beginning_ when I began experiencing sporadic hot flashes. This started in mid 2008. I would get flushed from time to time and thought I was having the real ones back then but, oh no, these were not them. These only happened once in awhile like once every few months or so. (Now remember, I'm speaking from my own personal experience. Women, your experience may be totally different.) By then my monthly cycle had already started to slow down. It would hit and miss, and by that I mean it would come every other month or skip months and come back. What I understood from my OB/GYN nurse practitioner was that I was experiencing peri-menopause, not pre-menopause, and that I would be in full blown menopause one year from the date of my last menstrual period. All of these other off and on occurrences didn't matter until they stopped for twelve consecutive months. So, each time I had a period I would start counting the months until my next one. Then I would start counting all over again. This went on for a couple of years. Each time they became further and further apart until finally reaching the one year mark. Even then I didn't experience my first real hot flash until about six months later. I kept having the occasional heat flushes.

THE HULK

Before ending this chapter, let me share one bit of information with you. Ladies, when you're having a hot flash, look in the mirror. I happened to catch myself in the mirror one day when I was having a hot flash and stared in amazement as my entire upper chest, neck, and upper arms turned a blotchy red. It scared me because I had no idea this happened when I was having a hot flash. It was a bit concerning to witness my body going through this chameleon-like transformation. When my hot flash finally subsided, my skin returned back to its normal color. What an eye-popping experience! I felt like the Hulk - only red! No really! Sometimes my head would even pound like a locomotive and my concentration level would decrease a notch or two making me feel senseless. Hulk, I feel you!

Remember in Chapter One, I mentioned some of the symptoms of menopause, which include headaches and concentration and memory problems. I have noticed that when I'm having a hot flash while having a conversation with someone, my mind suddenly becomes distant until their voice sounds like a muffled echo. Much like what Dr. David Banner probably experienced while he was being transformed into the Hulk, I can't hear a word anyone is saying. When it passes, I have to ask them to repeat what they just said. Now, depending on who I'm having a conversation with, I may ask them to hold on a minute until I'm done having my hot flash.

It also makes me feel a little dazed and disoriented at times, too, again like the Hulk. For example, in the morning I'm usually awakened out of my sleep by a hot flash. I figure since I'm awake, I'll take the time to go to the bathroom. When I get out of bed to take that first step, I start to reel a bit from being dizzy making me almost lose my balance. I have to stand still for a moment just to find my center of gravity or sit down to keep from falling. So, I've learned to just wait and lie in bed until it passes before getting up to walk.

I recently stumbled across a personal discovery that confirmed just how powerful these hot flashes can be. I was wearing my smart fitness watch for the first time when I noticed my BPM (beats per minute) tracker climbed from 65 to 75 in a matter of seconds while sitting still. I was also having a hot flash at that very moment and realized then that my hot flash caused my heart rate to escalate just like that. So, please take it from me - don't get up too soon from any position while in the middle of a hot flash. When you least expect it, it may knock you off your feet!

WHAT'S NEXT?

So, there you have it - my first hot flash experience, when the real one hit. In the next chapter, I will cover the _middle_ of my hot flash journey, and at the end of this book I will touch on what I think I know so far about what the _end_ of my hot flash journey may look like.

CHAPTER 5

FREEZING THE MOMENT

A HOT FLASH EVERY HOUR

So, after the first real hot flash at the upscale restaurant, I continued having them everyday. Remember in the last chapter I referred to this as the _middle_ of my hot flash journey. It started with maybe one or two hot flashes a day, which I thought was already pretty disruptive and intense. I had no idea what was coming next. Within a year or so, the intensity and frequency of my hot flashes grew until I was experiencing a dozen or more hot flashes during the day and up to half a dozen throughout the night. That's one every hour on the hour during my waking hours! They would come and go no matter where I was or what I was doing. And they seemed to last an eternity, but after timing them, they were no longer than a minute or two tops. That's long enough to be quite miserable. I had to find relief and quick! In this chapter, I will share personal techniques I've learned to freeze my hot flash moments.

TRYING TO COOL OFF

Finding relief was hard at first, but as folks say in real estate, - "it's all about location, location, location". Well, for hot flashes, it's preparation, preparation, preparation. I have learned to leave the house prepared.

In the beginning, when running errands, I learned to carry a hand fan. My favorite was a simple but beautiful oriental folding hand fan that a close Japanese friend of my mother's gave to me. I don't remember why she gave it to me. Maybe she saw me when I was flushing back in my peri-menopausal days. I carried this fan in my purse and brought it out whenever I felt a hot flash coming on. Yes, you can feel them coming. It's a surge that starts somewhere deep inside the body and spreads to the outer body revealing itself in the form of heat and sweat. You have about 5-10 seconds before you're rendered helpless. So, finding relief quick is an absolute must.

I remember shopping in a vitamin health store and had a hot flash at the register. Since the store clerk was a young male, I felt the need to explain my fierce fanning. So, I did in a motherly sort of way. He nodded and said his mother was going through the same thing. I smiled somewhat relieved, paid for my items, and then left the store feeling quite embarrassed. That's my earliest recollection of me hot flashing in public other than my first real hot flash. I can tell you endless stories about embarrassing hot flash moments in public, but I won't. You've been spared!

I wear prescription glasses and whenever I have a hot flash, my glasses fog up in the corners closest to my nose. Whenever people notice, they would point it out like I didn't know. I have taken pictures with my family and noticed that my glasses where fogged up in the picture. Needless to say, I am constantly taking my glasses off to keep them from steaming up and then wiping my entire face while at it.

I eventually had to upgrade to carrying a small towel, handkerchief or at the least a strong, durable paper towel folded up in my back pant pocket. The hand fan no longer did it for me. I would have to so fan rigorously, even switching hands, until it started to wreak havoc on my weak wrists. So, I ditched the hand fan. And besides, I found that unless I was standing directly in front of one of those high performing wind tunnel fans, having any other fan would be like poking the Jolly Green Giant with a needle!

FINDING RELIEF

So, the burning question, "What's my secret to finding relief for these never-ending hot flashes?" Three words - ICE COLD WATER. Stock it, travel with it. Never be without it. Even if, like me, you're not a big fan of drinking water, it is the quickest relief I know for hot flashes. When it comes, I have to find a way to cool my body down and fast! And a few gulps of ice cold water will do the trick.

I remember one time I was hot flashing so bad a friend got a cup of ice and slipped a few ice cubes down my back. I could feel the coldness of ice cubes as they slid down my back. That may seem like a logical solution, but let me tell you, it is not! For some reason, the ice was too cold! Maybe it was the shock factor. I jumped up and shook the ice cubes out of my shirt and let my friend know that that was not cool. All it did was make my shirt wet and make me mad. Needless to say, they never tried that again. So, as tempting as it may sound, I do not recommend ice cubes down your back.

Oh, by the way, modern medicine does not recommend drinking ice cold water either. It has something to do with shocking your body's internal system. So, as mentioned earlier, maybe substitute the ice cold water, with just cool or room temperature water. I have to be honest with you though - ice cold water makes me feel a whole lot better! It brings a sense of relief to my burning neck as it's going down my throat.

There are a number of other things that bring me immediate relief, which I have outlined for you below. The key word here is immediate. You DON'T want to be doing these things all day long:

- Standing in front of an AC or motorized fan
- Standing in front of an open refrigerator/freezer door
- Going outside if it's cooler
- Cold carbonated beverage (something with bubbles)
- Ice cream, sherbet, frozen yogurt, popsicle
- Taking a swim
- Tepid shower
- Taking off some of those clothes!

Do you want to know what else makes me feel cooler during a hot flash? This isn't exactly an instant relief mechanism, but if you have the time, it helps to watch a "cool" movie like "Life of Pi" - that's my favorite. Although this movie has its share of "hot" scenes, like when the main character almost dies from dehydration, the abundance of water throughout the rest of the film gives it a cool feel and makes me feel cooler. There's also "The Revenant" or "Ice Age" or "Frozen" or "Game of Thrones" - basically anything with snow or subzero conditions. So, keep this in mind when you feel like having a cool, relaxing day - do it with your favorite cooling off movie.

WHAT DO YOU DO?

There are some things I have learned to do and not do in order to live amicably with my hot flashes, which I will reveal to you in this chapter.

When I started having hot flashes on a daily basis, I realized they were not going away anytime soon. They became more frequent and grew in intensity. It was time to make a decision. Taking medication, for me, was out of the question. I remember hearing my mother decline the notion of taking estrogen and also heard bad things about it on television. That must have been embedded in my psyche because there was no way I was even going to consider it. I was down to two options - One, either living miserably with these hot flashes or figure out how to live with them. It was time to go to war.

My first step to becoming proactive was timing my hot flashes. This was really more out of curiosity than anything else. What I learned was pretty amazing. My hot flashes lasted about one to two minutes at most. The intervals between each hot flash were one hour almost right down to the minute. This was disheartening. Having a hot flash once every hour seemed impossible to live with. However, with this information I was able to pinpoint, to some degree of accuracy, when to expect the next one. This was especially helpful when I was outside the house and in a public setting. I could almost anticipate each hot flash and be ready for it.

Arming myself with the right arsenal was key. I mentioned the bottle of cold water earlier and also told you about carrying a hand fan or something similar for fanning. Another important item in my hot flash arsenal is the proper clothing. Wearing the right type of clothing that won't show disgusting sweat stains or cling to you like static - or I should say, a wet rag - is key to avoiding a hot flash disaster.

DRESS WITH LESS

Dressing in layers is a cool way to ensure relief. I go through great lengths to make sure I am wearing something I can take off without being naked. You laugh, but it's true. When you're having a hot flash, you really just want to be naked. Since that's not an option, in public anyway, I always wear a cotton undershirt or camisole underneath all my clothing. This is my first line of defense against sweat. Without it, I will surely be walking around with a big wet spot in the middle of the back of whatever I was wearing. I've done it many times and I've learned not to do it anymore. The second layer is the shirt, blouse or top I'm actually going to wear - this is what the public sees. Then I top it off with a light sweater or wrap if it's cool or bypass the third layer completely if it's hot. But that undershirt is the most important piece of clothing because it's going to catch that sweat. If it seeps through and makes it to the second layer - then better put on that third layer.

And, oh, very important - when leaving the house, make getting dressed the last thing you do before stepping through that door. Otherwise, you will be taking off and putting back on your clothes, which can mess them up before you even leave the house. Take it from me, finish getting ready naked or wear something light and loose until you're actually ready to leave. I have been dressed and ready many times to go out on a date only to have "melted" by the time my male companion came to pick me up. Then I have to take another few minutes to get refreshed or completely change my outfit. Speaking of melting, the "smell good" stuff we ladies like to lather on our bodies may be responsible for some unnecessary hot flashes. If you're like me, I love, love, love, "lotions and potions", however, as soon as I lotion up, a hot flash is soon to follow. This causes me to sweat in thicker layers giving the look and feel of melting. I suspect these darling lotions, body crèmes and oils temporarily seal the pores trapping in the heat. After melting a few times, I stopped applying lotion all over my body and now only lotion my feet and elbows. If you think about it, we lotion our face and bodies for moisture. Well, with hot flashes my body stays quite moist…

Getting back to the clothes, it is a process figuring out what to wear every day. It has been a major challenge for me because pretty much everything makes me hot. I've had to change my entire wardrobe to conform to these hot flashes. No more of my beloved things to wear like silk, rayon, chiffon, or even some polyester blends. I miss wearing my winter clothes like cashmere sweaters, wool coats, and everything suede and leather. I can't wear material that is thin because I'll sweat right through it and I can't wear anything heavy because it's too hot - even in winter. Oh, let me clarify. I'm talking southern California winter not North Dakota, Minnesota, Chicago, New York, east coast winter.

Another reason why it's important to dress in layers is to protect you from yourself. You can be so hot one minute then forget you're not going to stay this hot. Let me give you an example. I remember coming home from the movie theater one night and having a hot flash inside the car while parking. I was so hot I couldn't wait to get out of the car. Once outside, the night air felt great, but after my hot flash passed, I was trembling cold and had nothing to wrap around my damp neck. After going inside the house, I realized that was a good way to catch a bad cold. So, no matter how hot I may feel when I leave the house in the evening, I have learned to always carry a sweater or light jacket or some article of clothing that I can wrap around my neck. There's no sense in having a fever from a cold and hot flashing at the same time. That just wouldn't be right!

NO HOLDS BARRED!

So, being out in public is one thing - you have to endure your hot flashes with some dignity. Being at home is a whole different story because now you can let loose and just be yourself. You don't have to make excuses to anyone. Now, don't get me wrong - the hot flashes don't change. For me, they still came every hour on the hour. What changed was how I was able to react.

Oh, yes. Ready, set, go! I no longer had to be careful and behave like I did in public. When alone in the house, I can take off my clothes and strip down naked! I can open the freezer or refrigerator door (or both!) and just stand there for as long as I want. I can rant and rave, huff and puff, jump on the bed and roll around, turn on the fan full blast and chug down a cold beverage. I can do whatever I want! That's the beauty of hot flashing at home by yourself or in a private environment. It's no holds barred, ladies!

Now, of course, if you're not home alone, you probably shouldn't be naked, but you can definitely dress lighter. I also have a constant fan blowing, keep a slightly bigger towel handy, and have a fridge full of my favorite cooling-off beverage - sparkling natural mineral water!

GOOD NIGHT, SLEEP RIGHT

One menopause symptom I haven't touched on and really should is the topic of "night sweats," which are hot flashes at night. In the beginning of this chapter I mentioned having up to half a dozen hot flashes throughout the night. Aside from the obvious sleep disruptions, the night sweats would soak my pillow leaving it damp and flat. Ugh! My solution to that was to sleep with a thick towel on top of my pillow to protect it from my nightly sweats. So, starting fresh I began sleeping with a clean towel between me and a brand new pillow - changing the towel every night. Needless to say, I wash a ton of towels every week. As for the rest of the bed and my sleepwear, they stayed dry enough to get me through the night. Surely because I would kick off the covers immediately when I felt a night sweat coming and cool off before the sweat would totally saturate me or the bedding. As for sleepwear, cotton is the go-to fashion at night, too. Like the daywear, it works best for those sweaty moments. Definitely no silk or satin pajamas or sheets for this hot mama. And that's how I sleep right at night. Good Night!

STRATEGIC SHOWERS

You would think that taking a shower is a mindless activity. However, for a woman having hot flashes or night sweats, this mindless activity can become an event that requires thoughtful and strategic planning.

Depending on what daily activities I engage in or what I might have on my schedule the next day, will always determine whether I take a shower in the morning or in the evening. Without going into great detail about this mundane task, having hot flashes in your life can make a huge difference as to when you shower. For instance, after taking a shower, it takes me about thirty minutes to cool down. Seemingly, heat compounds a hot flash making it doubly hot therefore, taking an extraordinary amount of time to cool down. I call this a "double whammy hot" or *"hot on hot"* experience. So if I have something scheduled in the a.m., and decide to take a shower that same morning, I have to factor in an extra thirty minutes (sometimes sixty) to allow time to recover from any hot flashes before getting dressed. Remember, getting dressed is the final thing you want to do before stepping out that door. Or you'll need that extra thirty minutes finding another outfit to wear and change into. Something similar actually happened to me once. I had my alarm clock set for 5:00 a.m. to shower, blow dry and flat iron my hair. I had washed my hair the day before and purposely let it air dry that entire day and overnight so I wouldn't have to spend so much time under the blow dryer. My plan was to leave the house at 6:00 a.m. Did I give myself enough time? Absolutely not. I thought I did, but forgot to factor in an extra thirty minutes for cooling down after the shower, and in this case, I actually needed another thirty minutes because I was blow drying and flat ironing my hair. (As you will read in a few minutes, applying heat to the head while hot flashing is a super double whammy you don't want to rush through.) After suffering through my heat-riddled early morning rush, I ended up leaving the house at 7:00 a.m. - an hour later than originally planned. Did I make it to my meeting? Yes, barely in the nick of time, which is another "no, no" in my hot flash manual. Rushing to get somewhere will almost always bring on the heat or at least make you hot for reasons that could have been avoided if you had taken the time to plan. So, my fellow female fashionistas, add shower planning to the growing list of things to consider while hot flashing.

THE HOT WEATHER FORECAST

Living in a hot environment and having a hot flash can also be a double whammy. Another hot on hot experience. I'm talking about the weather. Fortunately, I live in a climate that is hot, but not humid. Here on the west coast of the U.S. the heat is dry. When it gets hot it's hot, but it's still pretty bearable because there's often a slight breeze associated with it from the Pacific Ocean. Those who live more inland may disagree with me, but that's the hot weather report for my part of town according to me. It's important to keep in mind there's not much we can do about the weather unless we choose to stay indoors where we can control the temperature. Having said that, if you live in a hot environment and you have a hot flash, things can get pretty uncomfortable fast. If you're traveling to a hot environment, you should definitely be prepared by packing enough clothes for any unforeseen wardrobe changes, like a mother packs a diaper bag to take the baby on an outing. She must pack several outfits for those burp and poop mess-ups. The key is to always plan ahead and *react* accordingly.

HOT HAIR BALLOON

There are a few more hot on hot experiences I can share with you. One is about hair - yes hair, the hair on top of our big heads! My hair is thick and fairly long. When I started having flashes I noticed my head gives off a lot of heat making my scalp sweat, too. This, of course, doesn't help when you have a full head of hair. It was very frustrating for me to style my hair the way I like it in the morning (using a flat iron for a straight look and hot curlers for a curly look) only to bundle it up in a ponytail hours later because it went limp or the curls fell from me sweating. I eventually stopped applying heat to my hair altogether and just started my day with a ponytail in anticipation of the hot flashes.

The real "hot on hot" with hair is the blow drying. OMG! Whether I do it myself or go to the hair salon, blow drying hair while hot flashing is ridiculously hot and has to be done in intervals. Thank God for the "cool button" on the blow dryer - that is a life saver! Even in a hair salon, an observant hair dresser can tell when a woman is having a hot flash and will immediately convert that blow dryer into a fan by pushing the "cool button" and aiming it at their face and neck. Amen!

Wearing my hair wet has become a popular go-to option. I remember wearing it this way all the time during the summer in my twenties and thirties. That's when the curly, wavy wet look was in style and easy to manage. I was tired of spending so much time on my hair because it always took way too long to wash, blow dry, and style. The idea of wearing my hair wet was inspired by a lady who rode the trolley on my way to work. Every morning she would get on the trolley with her hair wet. By the time she arrived at her destination, her hair had dried on its own and morphed into a beautiful do of big bouncy wavy curls. That fascinated me. So, I tried to duplicate her look. My hair did not respond the same way because our hair textures were totally different, but I liked the way my hair looked wet. So, I started wearing it that way on the regular, then went through a phase of not wearing my hair wet because I started going to the salon regularly. Now wearing my hair wet again is the go to, at least in the summertime, to keep my scalp cool during these hot flashes. Funny how things evolve.

TOO HOT TO TROT

Another "hot on hot" story is me working out. I'm not an athlete or even a person who works out regularly. In fact, I'm the total opposite. One could find me walking around the track in high school gym class instead of jogging or running. Team captains always picked me last for every sport and the list goes on.

In June 2011 I started taking a spin class after being diagnosed with gallstones. My doctor suggested I lose a few pounds before having surgery to remove them. So, riding a stationary bike seemed harmless and easy enough. After all, my sister and I rode our bikes everywhere growing up. Well, let me tell you, it was harder than I thought. First of all, I was 40 plus years older and umpteen times heavier. Second, I was sweating on top of sweat - natural sweat from the workout and ridiculous sweat from the hot flashes I was having several times during that one hour session. Needless to say, my relationship with the spin class lasted only four weeks and I don't even know if I lost any weight from it. (I did manage to lose 26 pounds in six months though by eliminating fatty foods from my diet. Yay!)

My point is, it's very hard for me to do any strenuous exercises during this stage of my hot flash journey. You won't find me making the rounds on the elliptical or stair steps or treadmill. Just walking on the treadmill works up excess sweat - let alone trotting or running on it. All I can manage for now may be 50-100 jumping jacks, 10-20 squats, a few leg lifts, or several lunges - and not all in the same workout. But that's the extent of it and that's not even on a consistent or daily basis. Oh, I do like to swim and the cold water certainly cools me off while I'm hot flashing in the water. In fact, I swam everyday during the summer of 2012 when I had access to a pool. After that, not so much.

HOT AND HEAVY

Let me just share this with you as long as we're on the topic of exercising and working out. Weight gain can be a valid concern for some women going through menopause. I know it is for me. Why do some of us have to be hot *and* heavy? What I don't understand and really want to know is why can't we lose weight with all this sweating we're doing from our hot flashes? You'd think we'd be lean as a string bean but the pounds seem to keep piling on no matter what we do or eat, especially in our midsection. I've gained 30 pounds since losing the 26 before my gallstone removal surgery. I don't feel like I've gained that much weight, but it's evident every time I pass a mirror. I look at myself and wonder, "Is that me?" Sometimes I'm unrecognizable to myself and have to honestly ask myself - when will it stop? How will I ever lose all this weight? It keeps climbing as time goes on and the older I get the harder it is to come off. So, I try to watch what I eat. Though not always successful at choosing the right foods, I try to minimize my intake and make smarter food choices.

My favorite sweets, sodas and fries are not good for me at all so I really have to stay away from these culprits.

No matter who we are, where we are, or whatever stage in life we find ourselves, we must take proactive approaches to make sure our mortal bodies are healthy, fit and strong as they can be. We have to think of food as fuel that our bodies need to keep it going. Have you ever noticed how much smaller the portions are that an elderly person eats compared to someone in their twenties? As we get older our bodies don't require as much food as a young person. If we want to live a long life, we need to take good care of our physical bodies. My late husband once said, "Why is it we always say 'look at that little old man' and we never say 'look at that big old man.'" He concluded it was because smaller men tend to outlive bigger men. That's something to think about. The average person doesn't normally see the damage excess weight is causing inside of our bodies. We only see the outside and want to correct that. Our inner organs, bones and cells need good nutrition, too.

There's lots of help out there for those seeking to make a diet change and/or supplement your body with high potency vitamins. It would behoove us to at least take a good look at our body, assess what it needs, and make those changes by seeking proper solutions to help our bodies achieve optimum health. I can't tell you what to do, but I can share what I do. I am a strong believer and advocate in supplementing a good diet with the right vitamins.

Currently, I am on an excellent daily vitamin supplement regimen, which also includes one specifically used for relieving symptoms associated with menopause like hot flashes. I tried it for thirty consecutive days and found it *did* help! When taken evenly spaced throughout the day as recommended, it helped to reduce the frequency and duration of each of my hot flashes. As for the intensity, it remained the same or only slightly improved.

I hope you find some of these techniques useful in getting you through your hot flashes and night sweats. Always think positive and don't be afraid to experiment and find more creative ways to freeze those hot flash moments! Then remember to share them with others as much as you can.

CHAPTER 6

95 AND FLASHING

"I'm 95 years old". How many of us can actually say that? Not too many and certainly not me. Only a privileged few have the honor of seeing this Happy Birthday come to pass. Can you imagine living that long? I'm in my mid-fifties and wonder what living forty more years would be like. Nice and leisurely - I hope. Let's see, I would be able to witness my grandchildren having grandchildren. How wonderful would that be? I would also want to be happy, healthy, and in my right mind. It can happen. I know a special woman who turned 95 this year.

THE MAGNIFICENT MRS. MAC

Her name is Mrs. Mac. She's keen, sprightly and a good friend of our family for decades who remembers details about us that I'd forgotten. Recently, Mrs. Mac walked the runway as a model for her church's fashion show.

The sponsors of the event invited her to participate and she had the support of many church members. Who says you can't be decked out in a Calvin Klein leather and wool accented suit with matching hat, shoes, and purse at 95? Well, Mrs. Mac dazzled like a diva in exactly that outfit and actually no different than she did in her younger days. Mrs. Mac is no stranger when it comes to fashion and was always magnificently dressed wearing quality, name brand clothing and stilettos that turned heads everywhere she went, even to this day. Just as she wowed the audience at that fall fashion show, she proved to us all she still has it!

Knowing Mrs. Mac has been a real honor and privilege for me. She and her husband were close friends with my parents for more than forty years. Her late husband and my father met before I was even born. Mrs. Mac has outlived her husband and both my parents. Since then, I have made it my duty to check on her everyday just like my father did when her husband passed. My parents lived across the street from Mrs. Mac making it easy for my father to see when she forgot to close her garage door before it got dark. He would call her every evening to make sure she was safe and in for the night.

As always, during one of my visits with Mrs. Mac, she caught me having one of my hot flashes and couldn't help but chuckle. She then shared something with me that made me gasp with shock. She told me that even at her age she has a hot flash every now and then that wakes her up in the middle of the night, and she finds herself kicking off the covers to get away from the heat. Mrs. Mac is not a negative person and would never tell me this to discourage me. She was just sharing a part of her life with me to identify with my hot flashes and I'm glad she did. This was good information to know. Now, I won't be so surprised if it should happen to me, Lord willing, if I'm blessed to live as long as Mrs. Mac.

HOW LONG ARE THE FLASHES?

So, I did a little research of my own to see how long these hot flashes can last in terms of years, and I found out that in a natural transition, they can last anywhere from five to ten years. When I say *natural transition*, that means menopause occurs naturally during the course of a woman's lifetime. I would be remiss in my duties as an author and encourager not mentioning two other ways by which menopause can be achieved, and that is *prematurely* and *artificially*.

"Premature menopause" occurs in approximately one in a hundred women. These are women who have an autoimmune disease, nutritional deficiency or chronic stress such as excessive athletic conditioning. This usually happens earlier in their life, in their thirties or early forties, and has a shorter duration lasting between one and three years.

"Artificial menopause" can occur suddenly and for a variety of reasons such as removal of ovaries, a cut-off blood supply to the ovaries, radiation or chemotherapy, or with the use of certain medical drugs that induce menopause for medical reasons like shrinking uterine fibroids.

LIKE MOTHER, LIKE DAUGHTER

You've heard of the phrase "like mother, like daughter." Well, there is a medical theory that suggests a woman's menopause experience could, but doesn't have to, be similar to that of their own mother. Wow, right? Well, in the same breath, they also imply that a woman's menopause experience is individual and does not have to resemble that of their predecessor.

When looking at my mother and her menopause journey, I wonder how my journey compares with her timeline. After having hot flashes for the past five years, I suspect that I could very well be following in my mother's footsteps with this long hot spell of mine. Only time will tell. I wish she were here today so I could ask when her's started and stopped. At this point I can only give a rough estimate. Let's see if I can figure this out.

I remember my mother had a miscarriage when I was thirteen or fourteen. That would make her forty-four or forty-five years old when this happened. My sister and I did not even know our mother was pregnant until she miscarried. So, her pregnancy may have been somewhat of a surprise to my parents, too. This means it's possible my mother was in peri-menopause or went into peri-menopause shortly after her miscarriage. I'll make this the starting point for my mother's timeline. My parents purchased an air conditioner for the house right about that time, too, indicating my mother may have started having hot flashes around then. After that, I remember her being hot all the time at least up until the time my niece was born in 1990, which would bring my mother's age to sixty-one. I realize this is a wide time span and may be off by a few years, but it's my best recollection.

Remember I mentioned muumuus in my Introduction? This could be an important clue, but I'm not sure it will help my calculations. My mother started wearing muumuus in 1976 or 1977 bringing her age to forty-seven or forty-eight, and she continued wearing them at least through the mid-1990's. The piece of the puzzle that is hard to figure out are the muumuus because I don't know if she continued wearing them for the hot flashes or continued wearing them because they were comfortable. This makes it difficult to pinpoint exactly when her hot flashes stopped. I'm going to stick to my guesstimate that her peri-menopause hot flashes started when she was forty-five and ceased when she was sixty-one. According to this calculation,

I can safely guess that my mother's entire menopause experience lasted for approximately sixteen years, give or take a year or two. So, if I am following in my mother's footsteps, that would mean I am getting close to the middle of my menopause journey if I accept my mother's timeline as my own. There are no two women alike, not even mother and daughter. My sister's hot flashes lasted for only a year or two. I hope she doesn't mind me sharing, but she also started her monthly cycle at the ripe old age of seventeen, like our maternal grandmother. I started early like my mother at twelve. Go figure?

Because no one can really know for sure, I can only hope that my menopause experience is shorter than my mother's and will end soon. In the meantime, I will let nature take its course and be thankful for my journey. The best part is being able to help other people along the way.

CAN WE LIVE WITH THE POSSIBILITY?

Going back to the possibility of hot flashing at 95, assuming we even live that long, the chance of still having hot flashes is probably slim to none. I believe Mrs. Mac when she tells me she still has a hot flash every now and then. But the key words to keep in mind here are "every now and then." That translates to me as "on occasion, once in awhile, here and there." I'd say having a hot flash at 95 would be a very rare, seldom or not-happening-at-all occurrence. With this in mind, I can live with that. If Mrs. Mac can live with it, then we certainly can, too, right ladies?

CHAPTER 7

PUTTING OUT THE FLAME

We have talked long enough about how *hot* these hot flashes are, etcetera, etcetera. Now it's time to put out the flame. The rubber meets the road in this chapter, as we address the following topics:

- Cures for hot flashes
- What do you take for hot flashes
- What you do when you get a hot flash
- Is there medicine for hot flashes
- Is there food for hot flashes

CURES FOR HOT FLASHES

Experts have made a big splash in the field of medical science when it comes to finding a cure for hot flashes and other menopause symptoms. They go back and forth between treatments like estrogen and hormone therapies being good for you one minute and then not being good for you the next. Penny Wise Budoff, M.D., author of *"No More Hot Flashes…And Even More Good News"* writes:

> *"Not only do doctors behave differently depending on who and where they are, but also women have different agendas. Actually, only 25 percent of the four thousand women who become menopausal every day in the United States and Canada use HRT. Most women want to take hormones to get rid of bothersome symptoms such as hot flashes, sexual dysfunction, and emotional problems, whereas most doctors are more concerned about osteoporosis and heart disease. It seems that women from different countries actually take hormone replacement for different reasons. Dr. Lila Nachtigall reported that 'French and South American women more often begin [hormone replacement] therapy to delay the effects of aging on physical appearance and also to improve the quality of their sex life. It was also found that HRT users were more likely to have had hysterectomies and were better educated and less obese than nonusers.'"*

Which is it? I'm not sure if they even know. Just like the egg. Remember the TV commercial that showed the egg being released from jail saying that it is good for us now after years of saying it wasn't? And by then, everyone had switched to eating egg whites? Well, just like the egg, the medical community appears to be sending mixed signals about the various treatments that may or may not work for relieving menopause symptoms including hot flashes. I could not find a lot of answers, just a whole lot of speculation.

For instance, some doctors believe estrogen is the *"preventive medicine that will decrease the morbidity and mortality of the growing number of older women in this country."* They are also confident that *"hormone replacement therapy has the potential to improve the quality of life and to prolong life."* Despite this consensus, the counseling practices of doctors in this country vary greatly when it comes to the use of estrogen treatment for menopause. It's no wonder many women still waiver in their decision to take estrogen when they reach menopause.

I learned some interesting facts about aging, particularly in women, that I am going to share with you. Did you know that women generally outlive men? Did you also know that women suffer more disability than men? And this is not because women outlive men. It's because women have illnesses that are related only to women. How is that, you say? According to medical experts, *"the sudden decrease in hormonal levels at menopause causes specific acceleration of some disease processes."* Wow, and I haven't even told you the scary part. Whether a woman takes Hormone Replacement

Therapy (HRT) or not, can still adversely affect her health. To clarify, women who take a stance and opt not to take HRT, for instance, may think that by doing so it will not affect them when, in actuality, it leaves them open to certain diseases like osteoporosis and heart disease. And even though taking HRT has been known to protect women, it does come with warnings of side effects. Then there's the natural route with herbal treatments, which can also be risky because many go untested even though the label says they're "natural." Even good old-fashioned exercise and too much calcium can have its consequences as well. So, what can women do to protect themselves through this aging process? The answer lies in becoming proactive in our own health care so that we can live long, healthy, and strong lives, not just for ourselves but for our families as well. We want to be there for them, don't we? And we want to be able to enjoy them in good health. Besides, if we don't take care of ourselves now, how are we going to take care of ourselves later when we're much older?

The main purpose of my book was to share my hot flash journey with you, but it is also my desire to give you as much relevant information about cures, medicine, and things we, as women, can do to help alleviate these detestable symptoms. Personally, I have not taken any hormone therapies or estrogen treatments for my hot flashes. Many women have been told about estrogen therapy by OB/GYN specialists. However, due to the uncertainty and controversies surrounding side effects and overall effectiveness of estrogen therapy, I chose not to take them. Was it the right decision? I don't know - but it was my decision. That may be why I'm still having hot flashes after five years and counting. But I'm okay with that as long as my body is healthy. So, keeping up with my medical checkups, submitting to lab tests, and maintaining an open line of communication with my health care providers are non-negotiable for me.

WHAT DO YOU TAKE FOR HOT FLASHES?

Nearly every resource book I encountered contained pretty much the same information as it relates to cures, treatments, and/or therapy for menopause symptoms. Even though I could not find any information that specifically gave an actual *cure* or *cures* for hot flashes, per se, there are a number of treatments and therapies that claim to have the ability to relieve or diminish the discomfort that comes with having hot flashes.

It is important to consider that everyone is different and there are no two women who are alike. So, it would be nearly impossible to develop one miracle potion or pill that will cure our symptoms. What we *do* have are choices. And that's what I will be outlining for you in the following pages.

WHAT YOU DO WHEN YOU GET A HOT FLASH

The first thing I would encourage you to do when you have one or more hot flashes is seek the advice of your medical care provider. Why? (Especially after all that talk I did about the medical community sending us mixed signals.) Well, first, I do have great respect for the medical community because they are trained experts in their fields who have spent countless hours studying the human body. They mend, heal, and save lives on a daily basis and, in my book, that makes them brilliant. Brave and noble souls are how I think of them because I don't have the guts to do what they do. Without them, we would be a hurting and broken society - literally. The second reason you should seek medical advice is because there are some other physical conditions that mimic symptoms of hot flashes and menopause, and you would want to be absolutely sure that what you think you are feeling isn't something else. A prime example that I found in my research is where a woman was misdiagnosed as "peri-menopausal and stressed" when, in fact, she had cancer. So, assuming you are truly experiencing menopause symptoms, there are some realistic and do-able steps you can take to combat your hot flashes and night sweats.

In addition to my own methods of "freezing the moment" found in Chapter Five, I came across this list of helpful things to do in a hot flash moment:

Self-Help tips for <u>Hot Flashes</u>

7 ways to cool down quickly

- Take a shower.
- Run cool water over your wrists.
- Have a cooling drink.
- Spritz water over your face or use wet wipes.
- Use a small battery-operated fan.
- Apply a cooled gel pack around your neck.
- Open your freezer and put your head inside.

Do not use cold or iced water. Both can cause you to overheat after you have applied them. Tepid water will evaporate on your skin, removing the heat, which will make you feel cooler and bring the feeling of fever to a more rapid end.

Self-Help tips for <u>Night Sweats</u>

Dos

- Do make sure the temperature of your bedroom is only 65 degrees Fahrenheit (18 degrees Celsius), which is sufficient for a comfortable sleep. If you have a fan or air conditioner, you may want to use it from time to time. Use a few lightweight blankets for flexibility.
- Do drink more water. You'll need at least 12 glasses per day at room temperature to cool down your core temperature without

shocking your system. Drink one glass before going to bed. Herbalists recommend adding 30 drops of sage tincture to a glass of water placed by your bedside. Simply take a sip or two as needed.

- Do wear sleepwear made of natural fibers only and make sure your bedding is also made of cotton or linen. Be prepared to abandon sleepwear; top sheets and blankets.
- Do shower or sponge with cool water just before going to bed.
- Do avoid all hot baths and showers.

Don'ts

- Don't do any heavy physical activity before going to bed.
- Don't eat before going to bed. Have your dinner several hours before going to bed.
- Don't drink coffee or alcohol, or smoke late in the evening.

I was actually guilty of doing a few of the "don'ts" on occasion and a couple of them pretty consistently. When I first read them during my research, I made a mental note to adopt a few of these tips for myself. This is still a learning process for me, too. I actually tried the "run cool water over your wrists" thing and I am happy to report that it worked for me! Who knew? I never, in a million years, would have considered doing something like that! Again, this worked for me and it helped that a faucet of water was close by.

IS THERE MEDICINE FOR HOT FLASHES?

"Medicine" is a broad term and I am not a doctor. In an effort not to appear as though I am giving medical advice, I will limit this portion of my book just to some of the "medicinal" options that are available according to what I learned in my research. Let me just say, for the record, that I do not condemn or condone any of these practices and that I relieve myself from any and all responsibilities associated with any adverse results that may arise from anyone participating in any remedies, treatments, or such like mentioned in this book.

I strongly encourage anyone who would like more information on any subject mentioned in this book to seek the advice of a medical doctor or professional. I cannot stress this enough. Your health is one of the most valuable assets you have and it should be treated like it's the most important thing in the world to you. Without our health intact, life can be difficult beyond imagination. Can you remember a time when you injured yourself in some way, and didn't that take precedence over anything else that was going on at that moment? You rushed yourself to the ER or

Urgent Care facility. Nothing else mattered - not work, dinner, or the kids. You had to get help for your injury! That's why ambulances have sirens and hospitals have emergency rooms. Commit to taking your health as seriously as you do your very life.

So, having said that, there are a number of remedies that may or may not help to alleviate hot flash and menopause symptoms. Among these are Hormone Replacement Therapy (most widely used), alternatives to Hormone Therapy (herbal remedies), and other supportive therapies such as acupuncture and reflexology. Within each of these treatment categories are many forms or types of treatments, particularly for the Hormone Replacement Therapy. As I mentioned earlier, I am not a medical doctor and not qualified to expound on different ways to administer these treatments. However, please make time to explore your options with your medical and health professionals.

IS THERE FOOD FOR HOT FLASHES?

Aahhh, finally, the FOOD. This is a category where we can all relate because everyone eats food. What can be said about food and menopause? A mouthful. What we eat is extremely important to our health and this is especially true during menopause.

What I learned about food and menopause is that there are menopause superfoods. Superfoods are certain foods that are considered a notch above the rest nutritionally. Here are some superfoods the medical experts recommend for menopausal women:

- ♦ Spirulina (fresh water algae)
- ♦ Wheat Grass
- ♦ Sea Vegetables (e.g. sea salt; Scandinavian purple dulse)
- ♦ Bilberry and Other Berries
- ♦ Maca (a tuber like the potato; has sweet taste)

NUTRITIONAL SUPPLEMENTS. Deciding whether or not to take nutritional supplements is another divided issue among experts. Some believe in them and some don't. Taking vitamin supplements, like everything else, is a personal choice and should be exercised with the same caution used for anything else that goes down the "hatch." According to some medical experts, the following vitamin supplements are recommended during menopause:

- ♦ Vitamin E
- ♦ Calcium
- ♦ Magnesium
- ♦ Vitamin D
- ♦ Vitamin C and Flavonoids

PHYTOESTROGENS. Now that's a big word. And why are we talking about it with food? Well, phytoestrogens can actually be found in several plants and plant foods. They are known as plant estrogens. They are structured like the hormone estrogen and can *"bind to estrogen receptor sites throughout the body, mimicking the effects of estrogen."* So, for that reason, phytoestrogens are considered a natural alternative to Hormone Therapy as well. This gives truth to what Hippocrates, the father of modern science, said over 2,000 years ago, *"Let food be your medicine."* The following is a short list of foods I found that contain phytoestrogens and are recommended by medical experts:

- ♦ Green soybeans (edamame)
- ♦ Canned soybeans
- ♦ Tofu or bean curd
- ♦ Textured vegetable protein (TVP)
- ♦ Soy & flaxseed bread
- ♦ Tempeh
- ♦ Isolated soy protein
- ♦ Soy flour
- ♦ Miso
- ♦ Soy desserts
- ♦ Soy milk

In my research, I came across some interesting data about the "benefits of phytoestrogens":

"Phytoestrogen-rich diets typically result in a 40-50 percent reduction in hot flashes, compared with a 25-35 percent reductions if nothing taken, and an 80-90 percent reduction with HT. While

the jury is still out on the subject of whether a phytoestrogen-rich diet can ease hot flashes, many women find it helps."

BONE HEALTH. When estrogen levels drop, so does the loss of calcium from our bones. This can potentially cause deterioration of the bones or osteoporosis. That's why medical experts recommend taking calcium and the following key nutrients during menopause:

- ♦ Calcium
- ♦ Vitamin D
- ♦ Magnesium
- ♦ Vitamin K
- ♦ Boron

On the opposite end of that stick are *"4 calcium depleters"*:

- ♦ Protein
- ♦ Salt
- ♦ Alcohol
- ♦ Carbonated drinks

Are you surprised? I am. I cannot believe protein and carbonated drinks are on the list as calcium depleters. We are told to eat protein because it builds muscle, blah, blah, blah. And now I have to rethink my favorite Perrier water!

HEART HEALTH. The heart is a hot topic of concern for people of all ages these days. What I discovered about the heart and menopause is that the HDL level in a menopausal woman can be negatively affected by the decline of estrogen being produced in the body, which can in turn put the heart at risk for disease. How can we protect our heart? Eating the right foods is the first step to improving one's health before resorting to medications. With that, medical experts suggest adding these heart-healthy foods to our daily diet:

- Fruits and vegetables
- Soluble fiber
- Nuts
- Soy
- Alcohol
- Cholesterol-lowering spreads and foods

WEIGHT MANAGEMENT. Now this is a heavy topic. Along with nutrition and food comes the subject of weight gain and how to manage it. Many women struggle with their weight even without the handicap of being menopausal. So, imagine how much more difficult it might be for women going through menopause. Not a fun topic, for sure, but one that certainly demands our attention if we want to lose that weight.

There are a couple of factors that can contribute to weight gain even before considering food as the culprit - the fact that we are getting older, which slows our metabolism down and fluid retention and/or bloating from some types of Hormone Therapies. Not only that, our body shape changes when estrogen levels drop causing fat to cling to our mid-section more than anywhere else giving the appearance of weight gain. As if this weren't enough, our food choices and food intake can greatly contribute to weight gain.

Managing our food intake can help us manage our weight. Let's go directly to the source. What is it going to take to lose this weight and to do it safely? The answer lies in being aware of your calorie intake and your energy output. The rule of thumb is to burn more calories than you take in. Some medical experts recommend the following guidelines:

> *"A woman's energy requirement varies according to her age, level of activity and weight. The estimated average energy requirement for women aged between 19 and 50 years is 1,940 Cals; for women over 50 the figure is 1,900 Cals. To lose 2 lbs. (1 kg) a week, you need to reduce your energy intake by around 500 Cals a day, which means that most women should be able to lose weight on around 1,400 Cals per day."*

1,400 calories per day! Are you kidding me? I'll starve to death! Can this really be done? Yes, you can achieve this by carefully considering your food source, reading all food labels, learning as much as you can about nutritious foods, and balancing them with each other to produce healthy, palatable meals and snacks. I am a believer of loving what you eat and eating what you love. Otherwise, it will be too easy to resort back to those bad old eating habits. So, finding healthy foods that look good, smell good and taste good are essential to eating healthy. I recommend going out on a limb and trying some new foods. You may surprise yourself and find something you like. *Don't knock it till you try it* is what my mother used to always say when trying new foods. There are some healthy foods that are actually quite tasty and don't have the look or feel of cardboard or chalk. Our bodies deserve to reap the benefits of healthy food. Your body will thank you for it later, if not sooner.

ON A PERSONAL NOTE

Before starting my research for this project, I often wondered just how much of a toll these hot flashes were actually taking on my body - from the heart palpitations to the heat surge in my chest to the pounding in my head and the enormous amount of sweat I was excreting from my body on a daily basis for the past five years. It's a little disconcerting when you take the time to really contemplate these changes and what harm they may be doing to your body. First of all, my body was new to these changes and second, these changes have been with me now for a very long time. If I can feel and see all of this happening on the outside, I can only imagine what must be going on in the inside. I've heard it said that as we age, our organs age with us. Think about it - this includes our heart, lungs, stomach, liver just to name a few. I don't know what's going on in there, but what the medical experts are saying about women and aging is concerning, if not a bit scary. I can't stress it enough, women, please take the time to give excellent care to yourselves - not just physically, but your whole self - mind, body, and soul. I'm talking mentally, emotionally, physically, spiritually and financially. I even include these in my prayers. Our body is a temple - not one to be worshipped - but we can certainly give it the attention it needs so we can live longer and look good as well. Am I preaching? You're right, I am. Only because I love you - all of you - you're gorgeous and beautiful creatures - fearfully and wonderfully made. That's us, ladies!

CHAPTER 8

LIFE IN DIFFERENT CLIMATES

Men and women are different as night and day - total opposites. By this time you might be thinking we may as well be living on different planets. And it may seem that way at times when it comes to these hot flashes. We may as well be speaking different languages, and most of the time we are because we really don't understand each other or what we're going through. In reality we're not living on different planets, but we are living *life in different climates*.

So far, I have explained what hot flashes are, where they come from, who they can affect directly and indirectly, what to do when they come, how long a woman can expect to have them, and some remedies that may help overcome them. In this final chapter, I would like to forge the relationship of the hot-flashing woman and her husband or partner into a happy medium, because, after all, she's hot and he's not.

HAPPY MEDIUM

When my parents were having their "battle of the thermostat" there was no happy medium *unless* one of them relented. It was usually my father who made the oven his best friend, but there were times when my mother would leave the thermostat alone, letting it stay at 80 degrees, and retreat to her bedroom where the open window gave her the relief she sought. As you can see, there was a give-and-take feature built into their relationship. That's what I think it's going to take in order for the man and the woman to "get along" during these hot flash moments.

PREPARATION IS THE KEY TO LIFE - OUTFOXING YOUR LIMITATIONS

Preparation is the key to so many areas of our lives. We prepare to go to work, we prepare our meals, we prepare our children for college, and we prepare for life's emergencies. Preparation, simply put, is planning ahead and planning ahead for hot flashes is no different.

When I thought about "preparation" and what it actually means, beloved TV actor Michael J. Fox came to my mind. Let me illustrate this point, if I may, with his story and bout with Parkinson's disease. I read in a magazine article many years ago that before speaking at public events, Michael J. Fox would take a strong medical cocktail just to get him through the event with minimal signs of discomfort that come with the disease like uncontrollable shaking, twitching, and speech difficulties. This was undoubtedly done to enable him to appear "normal" in front of the audience, perhaps in an effort not to cause fright or evoke sympathy. However, when he was away from the public and without strong medication, his symptoms were more pronounced and apparent. In other words, in the privacy and comfort of his own home with the love and care from his family, it was not necessary for him to be fully medicated as in public. At home, he was in a safe and accepting environment where he was treated like he didn't have Parkinson's. The medication for public appearances was something Michael J. Fox obviously chose not to take on a regular basis reserving it for those occasions when needed most. That took advance preparation. He *prepared* for these moments - he *planned ahead* together with his family and medical team.

(Michael J. Fox is a strong advocate for Parkinson's disease, and in 2000 launched The Michael J. Fox Foundation for Parkinson's Research.)

On a personal note, I am familiar with the harsh realities of Parkinson's disease. My own mother suffered from Parkinson's until she succumbed to it in her passing.

HOT-FLASH PARTY-PLANNING

As I mentioned in Chapter Five, there are some things we, as women, can do to prepare for a hot flash. It will take being proactive and consistent on our part. After all, it's our hot flash and we have to own it.

My days are definitely a lot better when I am prepared than when I am not. There have been times when I left the house without my cooling-off tools, bottled water and a towel, because I was either rushing or switched purses and forgot to transfer or include those items. In any case and for whatever reason, I neglected to take the time to prepare for my outing. On those occasions, believe me, I suffered. There was no water to soothe my burning neck and nothing to wipe my sweat. I had to hunt for a cool beverage or settle for a flimsy napkin, neither of which was usually handy at the time. Hence, taking the time to stop, think ahead, and prepare for relief can really save the day!

Making a mental checklist is something most women know how to do - the party planning type anyway. We can put our hot flashes on the party planning list. You know how we do, ladies. We don't want to forget or leave anything out and spare no expense! Think of this as your very own hot flash party. You can be cute and stylish with it or simple and sophisticated. For instance, if you prefer carrying a fan, whether it's handheld or battery-operated, own it - make it your own...outlandish and wild or plain and conservative! You can carry a designer towel or handkerchief or keep it basic white. You can have your own personal water bottle in your favorite color. Whatever your preference, you can make it fit you and your personality!

LET'S HEAR IT FOR THE BOYS!

Men, I'll keep this brief. You, too, can play a big role in preparing for a hot flash. I'm talking about what you can do to help your beloved when she's having a moment. Here are a few final suggestions to help you plan ahead:

- Make sure the fridge is stocked with her favorite cooling-off foods and drinks
- Know where to get a fresh, clean towel in a hurry
- Make sure the electricity is always paid up for the A/C or fan
- Remember, don't overdo it because that draws attention!
- A little moral support and good old common sense can go a long way.

Now that I've said that, let me say this. I know you men have a creative streak in you. I've seen it. You're innovators and inventors! You're planners and master builders! Let's hear it for the boys! I know if you put your mind to it, you can come up with new ways to make life easier for both you and your hot flashing soul mate. Coming up with new ideas for the family doesn't always have to fall on the woman. I know you already have a lot to do and think about. You're carrying the weight of the world on your shoulders, but please take time to interact with and love your family.

One thing we should start to realize, and some of us do, as we get older and closer to the "other side" is that relationships are the most important thing in our lives - not fame or fortune. So, our families should always come first, and guys, your wife should be at the top of that list. When someone asked Mother Teresa how we can stop the wars and fighting, her answer was simple and rings true. She said, "Go home and love your families." That's it? Yes, that's it.

MY HOT FLASHES TODAY

As promised, I will address my hot flashes as they are today. I'd like to say that they are slowing down. I feel a noticeable change anyway. Aside from having one or two *intense* hot flashes popping up here and there throughout the day, the duration and intensity of each hot flash has subsided quite a bit. Within the last month, I noticed they don't seem to last as long as they did before. For instance, a "normal" hot flash for me would last a minute or two. Now they are clocking in at less than a minute. Although the frequency is still the same, one every hour except at night, the intensity level of each hot flash has become less, especially at night. What does that mean? Could I be approaching the end of my hot flashes? I hope so. I think of them as my "mini" hot flashes now.

My night sweats have improved significantly as well. I think this has a lot to do with the room temperature at night. I was staying with friends who, for their own comfort level, had to keep the house at a very high temperature at night. I had to sleep with an absorbent towel on my pillow to keep from sweating it through. Since leaving that environment, my night sweats decreased immediately. I still have four or five of them through the night, but they're short bursts and aren't nearly as intense. My sleep is less interrupted and my pillow towel is no longer wet in the morning. I'm happy to say I'm feeling better overall.

LIVING IN HARMONY

Ladies and gentlemen, realistically speaking, I'm fully aware this may be a challenging time for you. When you live in different climates, life is not going to be fair for one or both of you. What makes it difficult is there are no real answers. It's like the woman is living in the Sahara Desert and the man is living in Siberia. They are worlds apart. However, there's always a different outlook - a different way of looking at things. Maybe we shouldn't look at relationships as give and take. That can be one-sided and lopsided. What if we upped the ante and started living our lives with a give and receive attitude? Sharing! Then we can live in harmony. The Scriptures say *it is better to give than to receive.* If we're both giving, then we're both receiving as well. That's a win, win.

I hope what you gain from this book is a better understanding of who you are, a newfound respect for your partner, and deeper love for each other. It's not enough that we live in different climates and that she's hot and he's not. The journey together should be cherished, remembered and hopefully shared with generations to come. So take *great* care of each other. Let's run this race together and win!

Acknowledgements & References

No More Hot Flashes…and even more good news, Penny Wise Budoff, M.D., 1998.

The Menopause Bible, The Complete Practical Guide to Managing Your Menopause, Robin N. Phillips, M.D., Consulting Editor, 2005.

The Menopause Makeover, The Ultimate Guide to Taking Control of Your Health & Beauty During Menopause, Staness Jonekos, Wendy Klein, M.D., 2009.

The Wisdom of Menopause, Creating Physical and Emotional Health During the Change, Christiane Northrup, M.D., 2001.

Menopause Perspectives Around the World, International Menopause Society, *www.imsociety.org*, 2016.

Government Approved Drugs for Menopause, North American Menopause Society, *www.menopause.org*, 2016.

BibleGateway, www.biblegateway.com. (Information taken from *New King James Version*, Thomas Nelson, 1982).

The Holy Bible, King James Version, Public Domain.

Langenscheidt's Pocket Merriam-Webster Dictionary, 1997.

Wikipedia, *en.wikipedia.org/wiki/Hot_flash.*

Google Translate, Machine translation site (*translate.google.com*), owned by Google, launched 2006. (Information taken from *en.wikipedia.org/wiki/Google_Translate*).

The Unexpected Route to a Spiritual Miracle, excerpt taken from *Tears to Triumph: The Spiritual Journey from Suffering to Enlightenment* by Marianne Williamson, HarperOne, HarperCollins Publishers, 2016. *www.oprah.com/inspiration/The-Unexpected-Route-to-a-Spiritual-Miracle.*

White Men Can't Jump, film, Ron Shelton, 20th Century Fox, U.S.A., 1992. (Information taken from *www.imdb.com*).

Me Before You, film, Jojo Moyes, Warner Bros. Pictures, U.S.A., U.K., 2016. (Information taken from *www.imdb.com*).

Life of Pi, film, David Magee, (Yann Martel), 20th Century Fox, U.S.A., 2012. (Information taken from *www.imdb.com*).

The Incredible Hulk, TV series, created by Kenneth Johnson, Universal Television, U.S.A., 1977 - 1982. (Information taken from *www.imdb.com*).

Michael J. Fox Life-Love+Parkinson's Interview 2012 with Ronnie Saddler at SN7 on YouTube *www.youtube.com/watch?v=vZQhpEgYM.*

Michael J. Fox Interview on Family, New Sitcom, Parkinson's - Michael J. Fox is Feelin' Alright After 20+ Years With Parkinson's by David Hockman, AARP The Magazine, April/May 2013. *www.aarp.org/entertainment/style-trends/info-04-2013/michael-j-fox-interview-parkinsons-family-career.html.*

Michael J. Fox Foundation for Parkinson's Research, Founded by Michael J. Fox, 2000.

Mother Teresa, Missionaries of Charity, (Information taken from *en.wikipedia.org/wiki/Mother_Teresa*).

The Revenant, film, Mark L. Smith and Alejandro G. Inarritu, (Michael Punke), 20th Century Fox, U.S.A., 2015. (Information taken from *www.imdb.com*).

Ice Age, animated film, Michael J. Wilson, Michael Berg and Peter Ackerman, 20th Century Fox, U.S.A., 2002. (Information taken from *www.imdb.com*).

Frozen, animated film, Jennifer Lee, Chris Buck and Shane Morris, Walt Disney Studios, U.S.A., 2013. (Information taken from *www.imdb.com*).

Game of Thrones, TV series, David Benioff and D.B. Weiss, (George R.R. Martin), HBO, U.S.A., 2011. (Information taken from *www.imdb.com*).

E.T. the Extra-Terrestrial, film, Melissa Mathieson, Steven Spielberg, Universal Pictures, Amblin Entertainment, U.S.A., 1982. (Information taken from *www.imdb.com*).

Strange Case of Dr. Jekyll and Mr. Hyde, a novel by Robert Louis Stevenson, 1886. (Information taken from *en.wikipedia.org/wiki/Robert_Louis_Stevenson*).

Jolly Green Giant, Mascot and TV brand, Leo Burnett (1935), acquired by General Mills in 2001, U.S.A. (Information taken from *en.wikipedia.org/wiki/Green_Giant*).

Calvin Klein Inc., an American fashion house founded by fashion designer Calvin Klein (1968), currently owned by Phillips Van Heusen Corp (2002), U.S.A. (Information taken from *en.wikipedia.org/wiki/Calvin_Klein*).

Perrier, natural bottled mineral water, Louis Perrier, France, bought by Nestle in 1992. (Information taken from *en.wikipedia.org/wiki/Perrier*).

Special Thanks

I wish to acknowledge and especially thank for their love and support

- ♦ My sister Sachi and niece Natasha, San Diego, California, U.S.A.

- ♦ My children Ronnie (Jeneice), Mario (Rose), Ronald, and Miki (George), U.S.A.

- ♦ My grandchildren Jalen, Brayden, Maurice, Georgie, Michael, Sydney, Tesia and Khalil, U.S.A.

- ♦ The Magnificent Mrs. Mac, San Diego, California, U.S.A.

- ♦ My Dear Friend Martha, San Diego, California, U.S.A.

- ♦ My Friend and Master Editor Sharon Hogg, Los Angeles, California, U.S.A.

- ♦ My Coach and Mentor Laval Belle, Los Angeles, California, U.S.A.

"For with God nothing will be impossible."

www.ingramcontent.com/pod-product-compliance
Lightning Source LLC
Chambersburg PA
CBHW060808050426
42449CB00008B/1595